AF412950

Horizons in World Cardiovascular Research

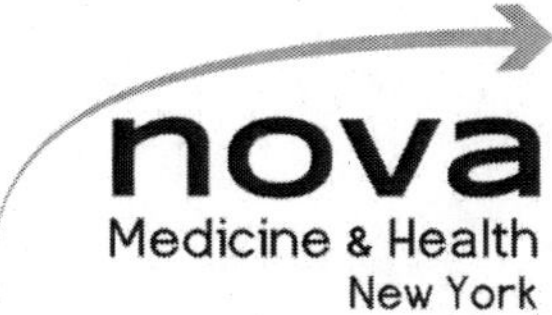

Horizons in World Cardiovascular Research

Horizons in World Cardiovascular Research. Volume 22
Eleanor H. Bennington (Editor)
2022. ISBN: 978-1-68507-568-2

Horizons in World Cardiovascular Research. Volume 21
Eleanor H. Bennington (Editor)
2021. ISBN: 978-1-53619-915-4 (Hardcover)
2021. ISBN: 978-1-53619-924-6 (eBook)

Horizons in World Cardiovascular Research. Volume 20
Eleanor H. Bennington (Editor)
2020. ISBN: 978-1-53618-310-8 (Hardcover)
2020. ISBN: 978-1-53618-360-3 (eBook)

Horizons in World Cardiovascular Research. Volume 19
Eleanor H. Bennington (Editor)
2020. ISBN: 978-1-53617-615-5 (Hardcover)
2020. ISBN: 978-1-53617-616-2 (eBook)

Horizons in World Cardiovascular Research. Volume 18
Eleanor H. Bennington (Editor)
2020. ISBN: 978-1-53616-925-6 (Hardcover)
2019. ISBN: 978-1-53616-926-3 (eBook)

Horizons in World Cardiovascular Research. Volume 17
Eleanor H. Bennington (Editor)
2019. ISBN: 978-1-53616-157-1 (Hardcover)
2019. ISBN: 978-1-53616-158-8 (eBook)

More information about this series can be found at
https://novapublishers.com/product-category/series/horizons-in-world-cardiovascular-research/

Eleanor H. Bennington

Editor

Horizons in World Cardiovascular Research

Volume 22

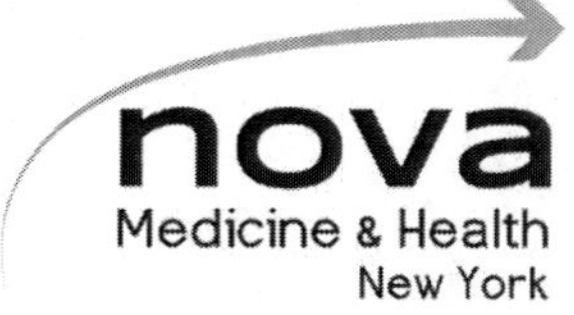

nova
Medicine & Health
New York

NOTICE TO THE READER

Library of Congress Cataloging-in-Publication Data

ISBN: 978-1-68507-568-2
ISSN: 2157-6130

Published by Nova Science Publishers, Inc. † *New York*

Contents

Preface

This volume includes five chapters that present recent updates in cardiovascular research from around the world. Chapter one discusses how histamine is transported from the gut via the bloodstream to the heart and puts forward novel evidence that histamine can be produced in the heart itself. Chapter two provides an analytical comparison of induced pluripotent stem cells, mesenchymal stem cells, and cardiosphere-derived cells commonly used for clinical cardiac applications. Chapter three compares outcomes of patients who underwent transcatheter aortic valve implantation with those who underwent sutureless aortic valve replacement. Chapter four analyzes changes in electrocardiogram leads, reflecting manifestation and development of acute and chronic myocardial ischemia. Lastly, chapter five reviews existing and upcoming cardiac magnetic resonance imaging techniques to evaluate systemic and pulmonary impedance in healthy individuals and cardiovascular disease states.

Chapter 1 - Histamine has long been recognized to exert cardiac effects. In the present chapter, the authors will discuss how histamine is transported from the gut via the blood stream to the heart but also novel evidence will be put forward that histamine can be produced in the heart itself, conceivably even in cardiomyocytes. Furthermore, histamine can be degraded and inactivated in the gut and liver but also in the mammalian heart. Histamine has been given as a drug for non-cardiac indications, but this was associated with cardiac effects in humans. Some drugs can release histamine from stores in the body and thereby induce side effects. Even histamine taken up by food can affect cardiac function. All known four histamine receptors (H_{1-4}) are found in the heart of some laboratory animals but also in humans. The main cardiac effects of histamine are species dependent. In humans, an increase in force of contraction and in beating rate is well accepted. Histamine may play a role for cardiac function in disease. Altered responses of the heart to histamine are now known in hypoxia, under ischemia, in allergic patients and in sepsis. Histamine might lead to supraventricular and ventricular arrhythmias. On the other hand, one can speculate that arrhythmias might result from histamine receptor dysfunction and therefore histamine receptor antagonists might be promising anti-arrhythmic agents. Histamine receptor agonists have been tried in acute cardiac failure in patients, though their benefit for mortality was never studied and they have not entered the clinic. In chronic heart failure, a blockage of H_2-histamine receptors might reduce the rate at which cardiac hypertrophy develops. Finally, various drugs also acting on histamine receptors, used for non-cardiac indications might affect cardiac function in beneficial or detrimental ways. These drugs include antipsychotic agents, anti-depressive agents, analgesics and psychedelic drugs.

Chapter 2 - Induced pluripotent stem cells (iPSCs) hold the potential to revolutionize cardiac medicine by supplying theoretically limitless quantities of patient-specific cell lines that can provide a more robust and clinically effective diagnosis or treatment. This chapter provides an analytical comparison of iPSCs, mesenchymal stem cells (MSCs), and cardiosphere-derived cells (CDCs) commonly used for clinical cardiac applications. The authors explore the utilization of iPSCs for cell therapy, including disease modeling, drug screening, and its potential for clinical therapeutic cardiac interventions. The economic, regulatory, legal, and ethical considerations surrounding the use of human iPSCs (hiPSCs) in the clinic are also discussed. Additionally, the authors delve into the current state of knowledge based on clinical trials and highlight gaps that serve as limitations against clinical applications. Finally, the authors summarize the outlook and possible futures for iPSCs in clinical cardiac tissue engineering (CTE) applications, which focuses on utilizing cells, growth factors, and scaffolds to construct functional cardiac structures that can repair or replace damaged tissues, arteries, and the heart. Despite their challenges, such as their metabolic, morphological, and electrophysiological immaturity relative to adult cell lines, iPSCs still provide an exciting and trailblazing opportunity to transform current cardiac clinical standards.

Chapter 3 - Aortic stenosis is the most common valvulopathy and a significant cause of morbidity and mortality in older adults. Surgical aortic valve replacement (SAVR) with sutured prostheses currently remains the gold standard of treatment for severe aortic stenosis. However, this operation may not be an option for selected patient populations. New developments in the field of cardiac surgery have led to the introduction of less invasive options for low to high-risk patients with aortic stenosis, or patients who are not candidates for surgical aortic valve replacement. As a result, transcatheter aortic valve implantation (TAVI) and sutureless aortic valve replacement (SU-

AVR) have emerged as valuable alternatives to surgical aortic valve replacement with the aim of reducing invasiveness of surgical procedure, morbidity, and mortality. The aim of this review article is to compare outcomes of patients who underwent TAVI with those who underwent SU-AVR. Study end points will include short and long-term mortality, postoperative renal failure, postoperative stroke, major bleeding episodes, vascular complications, paravalvular leak (PVL), cardiopulmonary bypass time and the need for pacemaker insertion.

Chapter 4 - While ischemic heart disease related mortality rates decrease, it still remains a major cause of death in the world. One of the ways to further improve the situation and decrease the mortality rates is the development of preventive methods and strategies, including early detection of ischemia. An attempt is made in the paper to analyze the changes in electrocardiogram leads, reflecting manifestation and development of acute and chronic myocardial ischemia. These pathological changes were modelled using ECGSIM simulation program. Its straightforward approach consists of alteration of the shape of the transmembrane action potential curve in order to obtain the corresponding ECG curves. The research investigated several areas affected by ischemia and three stages of acute ischemia development and a case of chronic ischemia. In all ischemia simulation cases information obtained from precordial leads exceeded those from limb leads and augmented limb leads. The most sensitive to simulated acute ischemia were precordial leads V3, V2, V5 and III standard lead. The differences in results obtained within the model and known clinical studies' results, are in the higher value of the V3 and V2 leads and lower value of V4 and, to some extent, V5 leads.

Chapter 5 - The rapid uptake of cardiovascular therapeutics and device technologies has led to a renewed interest in cardiac magnetic resonance imaging (CMR) techniques to non-invasively measure vascular impedance as an estimate of systemic load of the human circulation. Impedance, by definition, expresses the relationship between pulsatile pressure and flow in an artery. Cardiac magnetic resonance imaging can accurately assess structure and function of the great arteries, including flow velocity in the ascending aorta or main pulmonary artery. Systemic impedance can be estimated by ascending aortic flow velocity data coupled with non-invasively derived central aortic pressure data. In the case of pulmonary impedance estimation, non-invasive pressure measurement has not yet been demonstrated to be feasible. As such, a hybrid approach of main pulmonary artery CMR-flow velocity data and pulmonary artery pressure by invasive right heart catheterisation is described. The following Chapter reviews existing and upcoming CMR techniques to evaluate systemic and pulmonary impedance in healthy individuals and cardiovascular disease states.

Chapter 1

On the Cardiac Role of Histamine

**Joachim Neumann[1,*], Uwe Kirchhefer[2],
Stefan Dhein[3], Britt Hofmann[4]
and Ulrich Gergs[1]**

[1]Institut für Pharmakologie und Toxikologie,
Medizinische Fakultät, Martin-Luther-Universität
Halle-Wittenberg, Halle, Germany
[2]Institut für Pharmakologie und Toxikologie,
Medizinische Fakultät, Westfälische Wilhelms-Universität, Münster, Germany
[3]Landratsamt Altenburger Land, Altenburg, Germany
[4]Herzchirurgie, Medizinische Fakultät,
Martin-Luther-Universität Halle-Wittenberg,
Halle, Germany

Abstract

Histamine has long been recognized to exert cardiac effects. In the present chapter, we will discuss how histamine is transported from the gut via the blood stream to the heart but also novel evidence will be put forward that histamine can be produced in the heart itself, conceivably even in cardiomyocytes. Furthermore, histamine can be degraded and inactivated in the gut and liver but also in the mammalian heart. Histamine has been given as a drug for non-cardiac indications, but this was associated with cardiac effects in humans. Some drugs can release histamine from stores in the body and thereby induce side effects. Even histamine taken up by food can affect cardiac function. All known four

* Corresponding Author's E-mail: Joachim.neumann@medizin.uni-halle.de.

In: Horizons in World Cardiovascular Research. Volume 22
Editor: Eleanor H. Bennington
ISBN: 978-1-68507-568-2

histamine receptors (H_{1-4}) are found in the heart of some laboratory animals but also in humans. The main cardiac effects of histamine are species dependent. In humans, an increase in force of contraction and in beating rate is well accepted. Histamine may play a role for cardiac function in disease. Altered responses of the heart to histamine are now known in hypoxia, under ischemia, in allergic patients and in sepsis. Histamine might lead to supraventricular and ventricular arrhythmias. On the other hand, one can speculate that arrhythmias might result from histamine receptor dysfunction and therefore histamine receptor antagonists might be promising anti-arrhythmic agents. Histamine receptor agonists have been tried in acute cardiac failure in patients, though their benefit for mortality was never studied and they have not entered the clinic. In chronic heart failure, a blockage of H_2-histamine receptors might reduce the rate at which cardiac hypertrophy develops. Finally, various drugs also acting on histamine receptors, used for non-cardiac indications might affect cardiac function in beneficial or detrimental ways. These drugs include antipsychotic agents, anti-depressive agents, analgesics and psychedelic drugs.

Keywords: histamine, histamine receptor, heart, histamine synthesis, histamine metabolism

1. Introduction

Histamine was first synthesized in Freiburg in Breisgau, Germany, in a series of chemical syntheses of closely related aromatic molecules out of pure curiosity not knowing that histamine would occur in the human body or might act on the human heart (Windaus and Vogt 1907). These chemists sent samples of histamine to colleagues in Freiburg and Dale´s group in England. In August 1907, Sir Henry Hallet Dale attended an international congress of physiology at Heidelberg, Germany, and heard a young German gynecologist (Kehrer 1908) giving a presentation on extracts from ergot (secale cornutum) that potently contracted isolated cat uteri in vitro and Dale was curious what the active principle in this ergot extracts could be (Riley 1965). After some effort, Dale's group detected in ergot preparations histamine as the active principle and found it chemically identical with the reference sample from Freiburg (Dale and Laidlaw 1910). At that time, based on its chemistry, histamine was called β-imidazolyl-ethyl amine. The catchy name "histamine" to indicate an amine found in tissue (=histos ΙΣΤΟΣ) was coined possibly by Fühner between 1910 and 1913. Histamine research in the heart starts in earnest with treating whole animals (e.g., rabbits) with synthetic histamine and measuring cardiac functions including blood pressure in these animals (Dale and Laidlaw 1910). Dale´s group also studied the effects of synthetic histamine (prepared independently in England by Barger and Ewins 1910) in isolated animal hearts. Such studies revealed many observations that are still valid today. Histamine was shown in, for instance, living rabbits to reduce blood pressure and to increase the beating rate of the heart (Dale and Laidlaw 1910). In that paper, the authors speculated that histamine might mediate allergic and anaphylactic events (Dale and Laidlaw 1910). Positive inotropic and chronotropic effect in rabbits were probably first reported by Ackermann and Kuntscher in 1910 in Freiburg (Germany), and in more detail in a medical thesis of a medical student in Freiburg, Germany (Einis 1913). It was also noted that in coronary arteries from rabbits, histamine induced a vasoconstriction (Dale and Laidlaw 1910), but also a fall in peripheral blood pressure which indicated that the vascular effects of histamine are region specific. These authors also reported that synthetic histamine is practically completely metabolized in animal experiments (Dale and Laidlaw 1910). As early as 1913, at a talk given at our Medical School in Halle, Germany, synthetic histamine was reported to have been given to patients by injection and found to lead to tachycardia, palpitations (as a sign of arrhythmias), bronchoconstriction, reddening of the skin and a fall in blood pressure (Jäger 1913 a,b). Histamine as a possible mediator of allergic vascular effects in patients was suggested from clinical observations after injection of histamine in patients as early as 1912 (Kehrer 1912). Several years later, it was reported that histamine is not just a synthetic drug or present only in plants but can be found in organs of animals and can be formed in the living body of animals (Best et al. 1927).

Effects of histamine on the heart and the role of cardiac histamine receptors have been reviewed repeatedly (Levi and Allan 1980, McNeill 1984, Levi et al. 1991, Hattori 1999). A larger recent relevant review was authored by Hattori et al. (2017). In the present chapter, we will highlight developments since then. But for the general reader some background and seminal earlier findings will be discussed at least in form of tables. A very recent short review on histamine receptor pharmacology has emerged but the special cardiac effects of histamine were not discussed (Tiligada and Ennis 2020).

The effects of histamine in the heart can be differentiated with respect to species and with regard to regions in the heart and with respect to specialized cells within the heart. Interestingly, as concerns receptors involved in the cardiac effects of histamine, one can distinguish direct and indirect effects of histamine: in this context, we will address direct effects, i.e., histamine receptor-mediated and indirect effects, that are not histamine receptor-mediated but that are due to release of intermediates (e.g., noradrenaline) that then act on other receptors (e.g., β-adrenoceptors) or non-receptor proteins in the heart.

One even has to keep in mind also age-dependent actions of histamine in the heart. A didactically convincing example may be the chicken heart. In the embryonic chicken heart, the positive inotropic and positive chronotropic effects of histamine are mediated by H_2-histamine receptor and peak at 13th embryonic day but are absent at the 19th embryonic day (Tanaka et al. 1995). In contrast, in hearts from newly (2 days after hatching) born chicken histamine induces both positive inotropic and positive chronotropic effects via release of norepinephrine, which is obvious, because contractile effects of histamine were antagonized by β-adrenergic antagonists like sotalol or propranolol or reserpine (which removes noradrenaline from storage sites in the heart)-pretreatment (Tanaka et al. 1995).

2. Transport of Histamine

Histamine or its precursor histidine can enter the human body with food. Histamine is typically found in high concentrations in food which was formed by enzymatic processes: for instance, cheese and wine (especially red wines but with huge regional differences); in other cases, histamine is only found in food that was not properly stored and histamine content is a sign of food degradation by bacteria: fish and some sausages (Schirone et al. 2016, Taylor et al. 1989). The mechanism of scombroid fish poisoning was carefully studied by measuring an elevation of a metabolite of histamine (1-methyl-histamine, cf. Table 1) in urine of affected patients and it was claimed that scombroid fish intoxications are the most frequent form of ichthyotoxicosis worldwide (Morrow et al. 1991).

The cells of the intestine contain organic cation transporters which can mediate the entrance of histamine into the body (Zou et al. 2020). Histidine, the precursor of histamine, is also transported by more or less specialized transport proteins in the intestine (e.g., Bhardwaj et al. 2006). Some foodstuff contains large amounts of histamine which can pose problems for especially sensitive patients (Maintz et al. 2006, Schirone et al. 2016, Tuck et al. 2019). The increased sensitivity of some patients can have several reasons all of which are currently not completely understood.

Table 1. Synthesis and metabolism of histamine

Enzyme	Substrate	Product	Inhibitor	Reference
histidine-decarboxylase	histidine	histamine	α-fluoromethyl-histidine quinacrine NSD 1015	Jutel et al. 2009, Singh et al. 1999, Duggan et al. 1984, Levine et al. 1965
histamine-N-methyltransferase	histamine	N-methyl-histamine	quinacrine, SKF 91488	Yoshikawa et al. 2013, Sattler et al. 1985
diamine oxidase	histamine	imidazole-acetic acid	aminoguanidine, dihydralazine, chloroquine, tubocurarin, ethanol	Maintz et al. 2006, Sattler et al. 1985
diamine oxidase	N-methyl-histamine	imidazole-acetic acid	See above	Maintz et al. 2006
monoamine oxidase (MAO)-B	N-methyl-histamine	N-methyl-imidacyl-acetic acid	pargyline	Waldmeier et al. 1977
phosphoribosyl-transferase	imidazole-acetic acid	imidacyl-acetic acid riboside	FK866	Maśliński 1975a,b
alcohol dehydrogenase	imidazole-acetaldehyde	imidacyl-acetic acid	fomepizol, disulfiram	Maśliński 1975a,b
xanthine oxidase	imidazole-acetaldehyde	imidacyl-acetic acid	allopurinol	Maśliński 1975a,b
L-dopa-decarboxylase	histidine	histamine	α-methyl-DOPA, benserazide, carbidopa	Del Valle and Gantz 1997, Levine et al. 1965
diamine oxidase	histamine	imidazole-acetaldehyde	see above	Maśliński 1975a,b
xanthine oxidase	N-methyl-imidazole-acetaldehyde	N-methyl-imidazole-acetic acid	allopurinol	Aktories et al. 12. Edition
aldehyde dehydrogenase	N-methyl-imidazole-acetaldehyde	N-methyl-imidazole-acetic acid	fomepizol disulfiram	Aktories et al. 12. Edition

The synthesis and degradation of histamine was put together here. The enzymes involved are listed in the first column. The substrates and products of the enzymatic reaction are displayed in the second and third column. Typical inhibitors of the enzymes in the first column are listed in the fourth column. It should be remarked that the potency and selectivity of some of the inhibitors listed in column four are poor and whether they act only in broken cell systems, on purified enzymes or also on cells with intact sarcolemma or even in multicellular preparations needs to be meticulously tested. Some inhibitors inhibit more than one enzyme. Thus, the interpretation of data with the help of enzyme inhibitors should better be confirmed with, for instance, genetic models. It is also helpful to measure enzymatic activity in the cells of interest for the enzymes listed in the first column.

Table 2. Transport of histamine

Enzyme	OCT 1	OCT 2	OCT 3	VMAT2
substrate	not histamine	histamine	histamine	histamine
localization	outer membrane	outer membrane	outer membrane	inner membrane
inhibitor	quinidine, cyanine 863	quinidine	cortisone, decynium 22	decynium 22, serotonin
K_M for histamine mM	n. d.	1.3	0.64	4.37
further substrates	serotonin, dopamine	serotonin, dopamine	serotonin, dopamine	serotonin, dopamine

This table was intended so summarize our current concepts how histamine is taken up in non-neuronal cells with a transport system sometimes called uptake 2 (for a cartoon see Figure 5). The substrates are listed in the second row. Please note that OCT 1 probably does not transport histamine. The affinity which is quite low (but with a high capacity) for histamine transport (n.d. stands for "not determined") is listed in milli molar concentrations (mM). The location of the transporting proteins is given in the second row. Some often used inhibitors are listed in the third row. When preparing studies, it should be noticed that the inhibitors sometimes inhibit more than one transporter, are not very potent and have off target effects in isolated cardiac preparations. Hence, cell culture work might be preferable. Substrates instead of (second columns) or in addition of histamine are listed in the fourth row. (Data from Bourdet et al. 2005, Nagel et al. 1997, Gründemann et al. 1998a, b, Schneider et al. 2005).

What is clear is that patients who have low levels of the main histamine inactivating enzyme called diamine oxidase (DAO, produced in enteric cells of gastrointestinal tract but particularly in the small bowel) or monoamine oxidase (MAO, released from enteric cells in the lumen of the gut) are more likely to have high plasma concentrations of histamine and possibly cardiac side effects of histamine (Maintz and Novak 2007, Sasso and Perin 1999). Inhibitors of MAO-activity (like antidepressant drugs) or inhibitors of DAO-activity (like some antihistamines) would be expected to lead to higher histamine levels in the blood and in consequence in the heart and vessels. Indeed, aminoguanidine (a DAO inhibitor) increased histamine plasma concentration in psychiatric patients (Lindell et al. 1960). Most humans, however, show remarkably little side effects from oral histamine (Weiss et al. 1932), probably because histamine is usually so effectively degraded in the intestine by MAO and DAO. The main amount of histamine in the body is found in the peripheral organs not the central nervous system. Histamine is probably present (if sensitive enough assays are used) in all organs and cells of mammalians including humans. The highest concentrations of histamine are found in basophile cells (1-2 pg/cell) and mast cells (15 pg/cell; Jutel 2009, Shi et al. 2015, Knol and Olsszewski 2011). In mast cells (Ehrlich 1879), histamine is mainly stored in granules bound to anionic proteoglycans like heparin (Jutel et al. 2009). Histamine in mast cells was first described by Riley and West in 1953 and they reported high concentrations of histamine in mast cell-derived tumors of animals and humans (Riley and West 1953). Normal plasma concentrations of histamine in the literature vary greatly: in healthy humans, plasma concentrations of histamine are usually low, for instance, in one clinical study plasma concentrations amounted to about 10 ng/ml (= 90 nM: Coelho et al. 1991), or 1.2 ng/ml or 0.2 ng/ml (about 2 nM) and a range of 0 to 25 ng/ml with arithmetic means of 8.6 ng/ml and geometric means of 6.2 ng/ml in over 700 subjects have been reported (Laroche et al. 1995, Kaliner et al. 1981, Warren et al.1983). These large differences in histamine concentrations are probably simply due to different experimental conditions: handling of the plasma, addition of inhibitors of histamine metabolism to the freshly taken whole blood, storage conditions and unintended lysis of blood cells in the laboratory. In mice, likewise, low plasma concentrations for example 10 nM have been published (Ogasawara et al. 2006). The histamine concentrations in plasma are probably kept low because blood cells (for instance, basophils and mast cells) actively take up histamine (Othsu 2008). The plasma concentrations given above overlap with concentrations showing clinical signs of histamine intoxication: at infusion rates leading to plasma concentrations of 0.77 ng/ml (Ind et al. 1982) or in another study of 2.4 ng/ml volunteers complained of tachycardia (fast heartbeat, Kaliner et al. 1981) suggesting that histamine reached the sinus node and exerted here positive chronotropic effects. Besides mast cells and basophils in the blood stream, histamine can enter the vasculature of the heart also via thrombocytes. While the concentration of histamine per cell in thrombocytes is low, the sheer number of thrombocytes in blood leads to concentrations of 15-20 ng/ml in whole blood due to thrombocytes (Masini et al. 1998). Human thrombocytes can take up, produce, degrade and release histamine (Masini et al. 1998): release of histamine from thrombocytes typically occurs upon platelet aggregation by thrombin (Masini et al. 1998) and this might result in atrial fibrillation (see paragraph #13). Via H_1-histamine receptors, histamine, while inactive alone applied, can potentiate the action of compounds that increase platelet aggregation (Masini et al. 1998). Half-life of histamine in the human plasma is short: about 100 seconds (Ind et al. 1982). Human hearts contain substantial amounts of histamine, around 1000 fold more than the plasma concentration of histamine: in fresh transplanted hearts 5 µg/g of histamine were reported (Patella et al. 1995). Others (for review Wolff and Levi 1986) reported a similar order of magnitude, for instance, in human papillary muscles 700 ng/g of histamine (Eckel et al. 1982) which is in the same range as the noradrenaline content of the human heart muscle (500 - 2000 ng/g, Petch and Nayler 1979). Newer data using mass spectrometry basically agree with these older values. For instance, in mouse hearts (which contained remnants of blood) 10 pmol/mg (=1.1 µg/g) were noted (Zimmermann et al. 2011). Also using mass spectrometry, substantial concentrations of histamine have consistently reported in the human heart, e.g., in human atrium 845 ng/g (=7.6 µM) but also in adult isolated cardiomyocytes free of blood, at least from mice (Neumann et al. 2021b). At once, the question arises concerning the origin of this histamine. Some of the histamine measured in the human heart is thought to come via blood cells having been taken up for instance in the gut from food or produced in the stomach in enterochromaffin-like cells. In addition, histamine in the heart may arise from local mast cells in cardiac tissue (Patella et al. 1995) and there is a correlation between the number of mast cells (but also of cardiac ganglia) in the heart of a species and the region of the heart and the histamine content (Wolff and Levi 1986). Mast-cell-deficient mice contain less histamine in the heart, suggesting an important contribution of mast cells for the histamine content in the heart (Huang et al. 2002). On the one hand, histamine was detected in cardiac ganglia of mice (He et al. 2012) and men (Singh et al. 1999) and cardiac ganglia might thus also contribute to histamine content in the heart. Histamine can enter and leave mast cells and probably also cardiomyocytes by bidirectional transporters, called organic cation transporters (OCT) namely OCT2 and OCT3 in the heart (Gründemann et al. 1998a, b, Schneider et al. 2005) (Figure 1). In addition, in mast cells, histamine having reached the cytosol enters vesicles in mast cells via a vesicle monoamine transporter (namely VMAT 2: Travis 2009, Duan and Wang 2010, Figure 1). Histamine can pass the sarcolemma also by means of PMAT (Miura et al. 2017, Naganuma et al. 2014, Figure 1). Hence, cardiac histamine might have been generated outside the heart and entered via various steps into the cardiomyocyte. In addition, histamine might be produced in the cardiomyocyte itself by histidine decarboxylase (HDC) the main histamine producing enzyme. A next logical experiment to pinpoint the source of histamine in the cardiomyocytes would be to generate and study mice with heart-specific ablation of histamine production. This could be achieved by creating a transgenic mouse with cardiomyocyte-specific inducible knock out (KO) of HDC. One would predict no changes in histamine content in the heart of such mice, if histamine came from outside the heart or alternatively that histamine would be lacking in cardiomyocytes if all histamine in the heart were produced within cardiomyocytes.

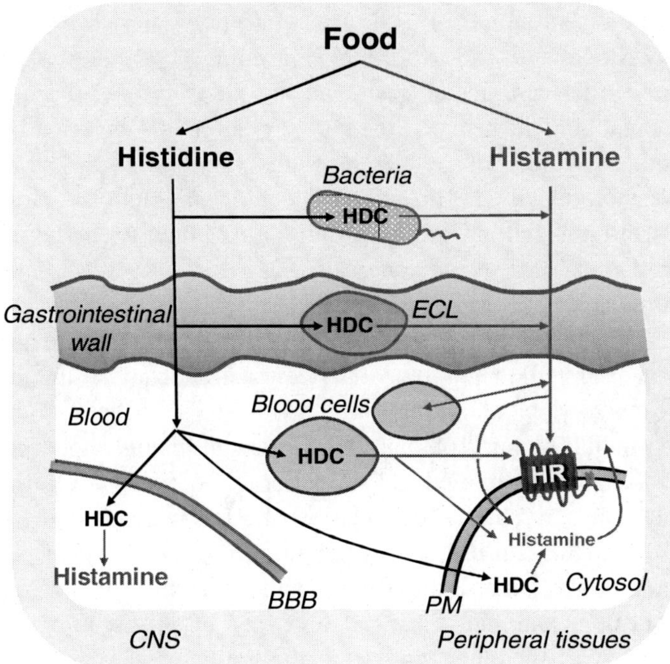

Figure 1. Intake of histidine and histamine.
Food can contain histidine and histamine. Bacteria in the gut that express histidine decarboxylase (HDC) can generate histamine from histidine. Different proteins can transport histidine and histamine into the enteral cells. In enterochromaffin-like cells (ECL) in the lining of the stomach, the body synthesizes histamine from histidine via HDC in substantial amounts. Blood cells take up histamine and enter the heart. Alternatively, blood cells may produce histamine via HDC. Histamine passes poorly if at all the blood brain barrier, but histidine passes the blood brain barrier such that histamine is formed by HDC in the central nervous system (CNS) and used, for instance, as a neurotransmitter in histaminergic neurons. Histidine can be converted in the heart to histamine and histamine enters the heart via blood cells. Free histamine concentration in the plasma is very low and its role, if any, is unclear.

3. Production of Histamine

Histamine stored in the heart can be released, for instance, by adding compound 48/80 to the Langendorff-perfused cavian (=guinea pig) heart. There is however a number of drugs that leads to release of histamine from cells to the blood plasma (see Table 3 for examples). Under these conditions, histamine is released into the effluate and can be measured in the effluate. This effect was more pronounced if the heart had previously been perfused with histamine (Pöch and Kukovetz 1967) arguing, both, for a formation of histamine in the mammalian heart and the possibility of the heart to store histamine reaching the heart via the coronary arteries. Compound 48/80 could also increase force of contraction in transgenic mouse atria with overexpression of the H_2-histamine receptor and human cardiac muscle samples from the right atrium extending animal data to the human situation (Gristwood et al. 1981, Neumann et al. 2021b).

In some cells like mast cells, histamine can be stored in vesicles. From these vesicles histamine can suddenly, following an adequate signal, be released in "bursts." In this way local concentration of 50 µM of histamine can be reached which should activate H_2-histamine receptors for instance in the heart. In the vicinity of mast cells even milli molar concentrations of histamine have been reported (Schneider et al. 2010). In a negative feedback loop, histamine can inhibit the formation of HDC in some cells (Schneider et al. 2010). For the cardiac content of histamine not only the synthesis of histamine by HDC but also the metabolism of histamine is relevant.

Furthermore, one can ask what levels of histamine are reached in the mammalian heart, in other words are the cardiac levels of histamine high enough to activate H_2-histamine receptors? Human ventricles after cardiac transplantation contain about 5 µg/g of histamine (Patella et al. 1995). This is about double the concentration reported in initial studies (1.91 or 1.00 µg/g: Anton und Sayre 1969). The cellular source of this histamine is unclear: mast cells were thought to be quantitatively the main source in human hearts (Anton und Sayre 1969). Consistent with this assumption compound 48/80, a known liberator of histamine from mast cells can release histamine from human cardiac samples and thereafter less histamine is found in cardiac mast cells (Patella et al. 1995). In mouse heart, lower concentrations of histamine have been reported, namely 0.29 µg/g (Anton and Sayre 1969, review: Wolff and Levi 1986). This was explained by low mast cell concentrations in the mouse heart compared to human hearts (Wolff and Levi 1986). A potential problem with these values is the presence of blood in the samples. In addition, the histamine content is usually higher in cardiac atrium than ventricle and this is explained by more ganglia in atrium and high levels of histamine in ganglia (guinea pig: Giotti et al. 1966, mouse: He et al. 2012, human heart: Singh et al. 1999, review: Wolff and Levi 1986).

Table 3. Effects of histamine in peripheral blood vessels

Species	Vasoconstriction	Vasodilatation	Reference
mouse: aorta	yes H_1? no?	no?	Van de Voorde and Leusen 1984, Russell and Watts 2000
cattle: arteria coronaria	yes: H_1		Garland and Kreatinge 1982
dog: arteria coronaria		yes: $H_1 > H_2$	Konishi et al. 1981
dog: arteria coronaria	yes: H_1		Konishi et al. 1981
monkey: arteria coronaria			Toda 1990
rat: aorta	yes: without endothelium	yes : H_1	Van de Voorde and Leusen 1984
rabbit: aorta	yes: H_1 (SMC, EC: PLA_2)	yes: H_2 (SMC)	Van de Voorde and Leusen 1984
Guinea pig: aorta	yes		Van de Voorde and Leusen 1984
Guinea pig: arteria pulmonalis		yes (EC)	Sakuma et al. 1988
Guinea pig: coronary artery		yes H_2: NO	Pierpaoli et al. 2003
cat: aorta	yes H_1	yes H_2	Van de Voorde and Leusen 1984
human: arteria coronaria	yes H_1 (SMC)	yes: H_2 (EC) cGMP H_1 (EC: NO)	Ginsburg et al. 1980 Vigorito et al. 1986a,b, 1987
human: arteria radialis		$H_1 > H_2$	Chipman and Glover 1976
human arteria mammaria interna	yes H_1 (SMC)	H_2 (EC) NO	Stähli et al. 2006
human arteria radialis	yes H_1 (SMC)	no	Stähli et al. 2006
Species	Vasoconstriction	Vasodilatation	Reference
human vena saphena	yes H_1 (SMC)	H_2 (EC) NO, PG	Stähli et al. 2006
rat arteria carotis communis	-	H_1 (EC)	Krstić et al. 1989
rat arteria renalis	-	H_1 (EC)	Krstić et al. 1989
rat arteria mesenerica	-	H_1 (EC)	Krstić et al. 1989
rat arteria renalis	H_1, H_2 (SMC)	H_1 (EC)	Krstić et al. 1989

The constrictor (second column) or dilatory (third column) effects of histamine receptor-stimulation, whether or not H_2-histamine receptors are involved, which cell type plays are role, the species and the vessel studied (first column) are listed for comparison. From this table, it can be concluded that translation from animal vessels to human vessels is not a trivial question. SMC: smooth muscle cells. EC: endothelial cells. "yes" or "no" are intended to indicate that vasoconstriction or vasodilatation was reported in the paper listed in the fourth column. NO or PG mean that the dilatation is known to be mediated by nitric oxide or prostaglandins. "cGMP" means that the involvement of an increase in cGMP initiates the vasodilation (see also Figure 4). H_1 and H_2 indicate the involvement of H_1-histamine receptors or H_2-histamine receptors.

As just mentioned, histamine can be formed mainly if not solely by histidine decarboxylase (HDC, Werle 1936) in all cells that contain HDC as a protein after translation. HDC is targeted to the endoplasmic reticulum where it undergoes partial proteolysis to a more active form in granules (Ichikawa et al. 2010). In mast cells, the synthesis of histamine via HDC is induced by glucocorticoids (Ichikawa et al. 2010). Histamine is then formed from histidine in the cytosol of the cell and can be pumped into vesicles. From these vesicles upon stimuli large amounts of histamine are released via degranulation, in, for instance, mast cells or neutrophils, leading to high local histamine concentrations (Ichikawa et al. 2010). Such granules are lacking in many other cells, like cardiomyocytes. In non-mast cells histamine is thought to be continuously formed by cytosolic HDC and histamine is thought to be continuously released from the producing cell with the help of OCTs (Ichikawa et al. 2010).

Currently, there is much interest on the so called microbiome in the intestinal tract (Pugin and Barcik 2017). A third of the metabolism of histidine by means of HDC to histamine in the human body seems to occur by microorganisms in the gastrointestinal tract (Frei et al. 2014). Normal Escherichia coli-bacteria do not contain HDC activity, but other bacteria in the human gastrointestinal tract are known to have highly active HDC and this varies interindividually (Pugin and Barcik 2017). Bacteria also produce via HDC new histamine in foodstuff like wine and cheese which can lead to cardiac events like arrhythmias (Ferstl et al. 2014). Moreover, in some asthmatic patients, bacteria in the lung contain more HDC and thus are more likely to produce histamine than in healthy humans (Barcik et al. 2017). Histamine formed in this way in the lung is also expected to reach the circulation. Thus, many cells in or on the human body can form histamine to an unpredictable extent. In our context, it is relevant that probably all cell types normally present in the mammalian heart can form histamine. It is noteworthy that histamine can be formed probably also in the mouse and human heart: HDC could be detected in isolated ventricular cardiomyocytes from adult mice in Western blots and using immunohistochemistry in ventricular cardiomyocytes from adult mice and adult human atrial samples (Neumann et al. 2021).

There are a number of known mutations of HDC, some of which lead to reduced activity of HDC (Ercan-Sensicek et al. 2010). Whether these patients have less histamine in the heart has apparently not yet reported but would be predicted. Histidine, at high concentrations, can elicit a positive inotropic effect in the human heart (Neumann et al. 2021), suggesting that histidine can be metabolized by HDC to histamine which then acts on the surface of the cardiomyocytes on, for instance, sarcolemmal H_2-histamine receptors. At least in salivary gland cells local histamine concentrations at the outer cell membrane can reach up to 50 μM (Stegaev et al. 2013). It is unclear, whether such high local concentrations of histamine are reached near cardiomyocytes. In addition, a well-known source of cardiac histamine resides in mast cells: mast cells can form histamine and release histamine which then can activate histamine receptors. In the vicinity of mast cells very high concentrations of histamine up to mM are expected (Hirasawa 2019). Released histamine should act at the histamine receptor most adjacent to mast cells but in addition histamine is expected to bind to histamine receptors with the highest affinity and then to lower affinity and so on. That means histamine is expected first to bind (and activate) H_4, H_3, H_1- and lastly H_2-histamine receptors (see Table 1). It might merit mentioning that in many diseased states the concentration of mast cells increases in the heart, for instance it some forms of heart failure (Patella et al. 1998) but also in some forms of generalized mastocytosis (Rohr et al. 2005, Shaffer et al. 2006). There are in vitro data that L-Dopa decarboxylase (Table 3), the enzyme that produces dopamine and which is present also in the heart can generate histamine from histidine (Levine 1965, Del Valle and Gantz 1997). In contrast, it was reported that in the blood plasma of patients suffering from Parkinson's disease, histamine levels are lower after they received L-dopa and carbidopa, an enzyme that inhibits L-Dopa decarboxylase activity, compared to controls (Coelho et al. 1991). However, the role of L-Dopa decarboxylase for the production of histamine in the heart remains uncertain but could be resolved by using knock out mice (see below) which apparently has not yet been reported.

The expression of HDC and therefore the histamine production can be increased and decreased by chemical compounds. For instance, dexamethasone (a glucocorticoid), can induce the expression of HDC in mastocytoma cells (Imanishi et al. 1987). Injection of interleukin-1, tumor necrosis factor α or of lipopolysaccharides (= LPS) into animals will increase the expression HDC (in the stomach: Endo and Kumagai 1998, in the liver: Neugebauer et al. 2004; lung and kidney: Hattori et al. 2016) and also in the heart (rabbit atrium: Matsuda et al. 2002). Thyrotropic hormone, injected in living rats was reported to increase HDC activity in their hearts (Lorenz et al. 1968). In general, during infectious diseases via cytokines will increase the expression and activity of HDC and thus histamine formation (review: Moriguchi and Takai 2020). This induction of HDC and increase in histamine levels also occurs in mast-cell deficient mice, suggesting the mast cells are not the only cell type where LPS induces HDC but this induction occurs in several cell types (Endo et al. 1995). Interestingly, endurance exercise in mice for more than two hours increased the expression of HDC in skeletal muscle (Niijima-Yaoita et al. 2012): one might speculate that cardiac exercise has a similar effect, but this has not yet been reported. The promoter of the HDC gene is activated in vitro by phorbol esters, cAMP-derivatives in the presence of elevated Ca^{2+} or oxidative stress (Höcker et al. 1998, Ichikawa et al. 2010) This may explain the effect of LPS or ischemia on histamine levels (see paragraph #10-12). If however, HDC is already disease-related elevated, then dexamethasone can reduce HDC expression (nasal mucosa: Kitamura et al. 2006). The exact underlying mechanism(s) for promoter activity of HDC in sepsis are currently the subject of active research (Takai et al. 2019). In cardiac sympathetic nerve endings (synaptosomes), a similar pathway was detected: L-histidine or quinacrine treatment (each alone or together) increased the amount of released histamine by depolarization in the synaptosomes (Li et al. 2006). Mast cells can release histamine in an immunologically induced way or in a non-immunologically induced way (Table 3). A non-immunologically way is the release by low temperatures. There are subjects that develop in cold or congelation surroundings (or in cold water) a so called cold urticaria where the skin is red and shows weals. In such patients, rapid increases in plasma histamine were reported and it is thought that their symptoms are at least in part mediated by this plasma histamine acting on histamine receptors (Dyer et al. 1982).

4. Degradation of Histamine

In principle, it was already shown in one of the initial papers on histamine, that the isolated perfused liver of animals nearly completely metabolizes histamine and that orally applied histamine in animals leaves the body nearly solely as degradation products (Dale and Laidlaw 1910). Histamine can in principle be metabolized by several enzymes: one such pathway is initiated by histaminylation by means of a transglutaminase (Wajda et al. 1961). Possibly also relevant in cardiac sepsis: LPS could increase transglutaminase activity and hence could reduce the level of histamine in the heart (and other organs). Interestingly, transglutamination is apparently not simply a mode to get rid of histamine for the cell but can alter the activity of some very important signal transduction molecules: histaminylation of G-proteins was reported to alter their enzymatic activity (Walther et al. 2011, Vowinckel et al. 2012). Histaminylation alters the function of fibrinogen, thus one might regard histamine as a second messenger (Lai and Greenberg 2013, Walther et al.

2011). The presence of histaminylation in the heart has apparently not been yet reported.

Another pathway for (extracellular) histamine degradation is based on DAO. This enzyme is not specific for histamine, but as its name implies will metabolizes many amines. Most DAO is formed in the liver, can leave the liver, enters the blood stream and by this way keeps plasma histamine concentrations low (Maintz et al. 2006). In man (and mice), only one isoenzyme of diaminoxidase has been found so far (Schwelberger et al. 2013, 2018). Some investigators found in mouse cardiomyocytes very little if any DAO, whereas in mouse cardiac endothelial cells, DAO was present (Bono et al. 1999). In the porcine heart, no activity of DAO was measurable (Klocker et al. 2005). It might be of clinical interest that in animal experiments, heparin could release histamine-N-methyltransferase (HMT) from endothelial cells which would be expected to reduce cardiac levels of histamine. Histamine increased the plasma activity of DAO and this might be negative feedback loop (Wollin et al. 1998). DAO activity can be reduced by drugs like dihydralazine, chloroquine, cycloserine, tubocurarin, cimetidine, dihydralazine and diphenhydramine (Sattler et al. 1985, Wantke et al. 1998). Through this indirect interaction, these drugs might elevate histamine levels and could induce, for instance, cardiac arrhythmias (see paragraph #13). Some polymorphisms of DAO have reduced enzymatic activity and have been correlated with gut diseases like Crohn's disease or food induced allergy, as they will increase histamine levels (Maintz et al. 2006, Jones and Kearns 2011). More important in our context is that DAO activity was found increased in patients with heart failure and was a negative predictor of survival (Boomsma et al. 1997). DAO is mainly responsible for inactivation of histamine taken in by food because it is found in cells in the gastrointestinal tract and is constantly released into the lumen of the gut where it can inactivate histamine present in food or degrade histamine formed by bacteria in the gut (Sattler et al. 1988). It might be of value to remember that alcoholic beverages inhibit the activity of DAO and this might explain some untoward effects of alcohol in selected patients (Dzudie et al. 2018). Moreover, 1-methyl-histamine formed from histamine by HMT (Table 1), is further degraded by monoamine oxidase B (MAO-B, also immunologically present in human heart: Duicu et al. 2015) in the outer membranes of mitochondria (Waldmeier et al. 1977). This is leads to the formation of H_2O_2 which is known to be involved in the genesis of cardiac hypertrophy (Kaludercic et al. 2011). The various metabolic steps mentioned above (see Table 1 for details) are so effective that less than 3% of exogenously applied histamine is recovered in urine (Maśliński 1975a, b, Kaliner et al. 1982).

Histamine entering the heart via the blood or formed in the heart can leave the heart unaltered via the blood. However, there is evidence that histamine can also be metabolized in the heart: the enzymes responsible for metabolism can be detected histo-immunologically in samples of human (also mouse and pig) hearts. When the metabolizing enzymes are inhibited by drugs, the positive inotropic effects of histamine are potentiated, suggesting that the metabolism is fast and effective enough to alter histamine levels near the H_2-histamine receptors on cardiomyocytes (Neumann et al. 2021). Inhibition of MAO-B should increase the level of histamine and therefore increase functional effects of exogenous or endogenous histamine on cardiac histamine receptors. When interpreting murine studies, one has to keep in mind that rats preferentially exhibit MAO-A activity and mice MAO-B activity in the heart (Dorris 1982, Kaludercic et al. 2010). In human hearts, in contrast, about equal levels of expression of MAO-A and MAO-B were reported (Duicu et al. 2015). Clinically, tranylcypromine (an antidepressant that inhibits irreversibly both MAO-A and MAO-B) or selegiline (used to treat Parkinson's disease and preferentially inhibiting irreversibly MAO-B) are expected to increase the plasma concentrations of histamine and thus the incidence of histamine mediated arrhythmias in these patients. This might be especially relevant in the elderly: they are prone to suffer both from Parkinson's disease and atrial fibrillation. For instance, register studies are needed to prove this hypothesis. Initial data are present from rats: here tranylcypromine and selegiline increased the concentrations of histamine in the urine if animals were given orally radioactive histamine before (Benedetti et al. 1980). Metabolism of histamine in the heart seems to be affected in part by diamine oxidase (DAO, also known as histaminase (Table 1)), because it was inhibited by aminoguanidine in a transgenic mouse model that overexpressed human H_2-histamine receptors and DAO was enzymatically, histologically and using Western blotting detectable in the human heart (Neumann et al. 2021). Typically, DAO is regarded as a secretable enzyme present in plasma and the lumen of the gut (Maintz et al. 2006). It may be secreted from endothelial cells on the vessel wall and might thereby contribute to low histamine levels in the plasma (Schwelberger 2013, 2018). Polymorphisms of DAO with reduced enzyme activity are known but cardiac consequences have not been studied in detail (Jones and Kearns 2011). DAO-inhibition by aminoguanidine in vivo leads to tachycardia: pigs treated orally with 50 mg histamine had normal heart rate, but when aminoguanidine was also applied tachycardia ensued (Sattler et al. 1988) suggesting a role of DAO for cardiac histamine levels. In addition, in some forms of heart failure increased DAO activity was noted (Boosma et al. 1997). This could be a compensatory mechanism as elevated levels of histamine in heart failure were reported (Boosma et al. 1997). Humans seem to be usually quite resilient against histamine: 500 mg histamine per os did not induce tachycardia in a study (Weiss et al. 1932) Moreover, HMT probably is also relevant in the human heart, because it was detectable in human cardiomyocytes using immunohistochemistry, using Western blotting (in mouse and human heart) and enzymatically (in mouse heart and human heart) (Bono et al. 1999, Neumann et al. 2021a). Interestingly, DAO seems to be mainly located in plasma and seems to be responsible, in part, to keep histamine concentrations low in the blood. In the heart, it is conceivable that DAO, located on the outer surface of cardiovascular cells, reduces histamine concentrations in the vicinity of sarcolemma histamine receptors and in this was attenuates histamine receptor mediated effects. Drinking histamine rich red wine led to transient increases in plasma activity of DAO in healthy volunteers (Wantke et al. 1999). As mentioned above, in the porcine heart, no DAO was detectable indicating that species differences in histamine metabolism in the heart exist (Klocker et al. 2005). DAO is also present in proximal tubular cells and also histamine-N-methyltransferase was found in the kidney (Schwelberger et al. 2013, 2018). One metabolite of histamine is imidazol-4-acetic acid which in the brain binds probably to imidazoline-receptors: these receptors have also been described in the heart (Maltsev et al. 2014, Preuss et al. 1997): the physiological cardiac relevance, if any, of this pathway is currently unclear. Isoproterenol subcutaneously given to induce reversible cardiac hypertrophy in rats, led in the heart to a reversible increase in the activity of DAO (Perin et al. 1983).

The situation for HMT is also complicated. At least in the kidney, HMT is present mainly if not exclusively in the cytosol of kidney cells (Grange et al. 2019). Hence, histamine formed in cardiomyocytes via HDC would be at once degraded by HMT in cardiomyocytes. After β_2-adrenoceptor stimulation in transfected HEK cells, HMT can translocate to the membranes of cells but would remain in the cytosol and degrade histamine just below the cell membrane (Ogasawara et al. 2006). Thus, one has to assume different subcellular compartments of HDC and HMT in cardiomyocytes to explain the quite high intracellular histamine concentrations in cardiomyocytes. More work is needed to resolve this issue.

Table 4. Histamine-receptors

Receptor	H$_1$	H$_2$	H$_3$	H$_4$	Reference
Affinity K$_D$ values	160 nM	1 µM	40 nM	30 nM	Seifert et al. 2013
Agonist	histamine, 2-methyl-histamine, 2-pyridyl-ethylamine	histamine, impromidine, 4-methyl-histamine dimaprit	histamine, imetit, R-α-methyl-histamine, methimepip, N^α-methyl-histamine, immepip	histamine dimaprit, 4-methyl-histamine JNJ28610244, imetit, R-α-methyl-histamine, immepip, clobenpropit, immethridine	Tillgada and Ennis 2020, Kitbunnadaj et al. 2004
Antagonist	mepyramine (=pyrilamine), diphen-hydramine	burimamide, cimetidine, famotidine, tiotidine, metiamide	thioperamide, pitolisant, JNJ52076852, clobenpropit, ciproxifan, burimamide, amiodarone, lorcainide	JNJ7777120, A943931	Del Tredici et al. 2013
cAMP-level	reduced via Gi/o	increased Via Gs	reduced via Gi/o	reduced via Gi/o	
	IP$_3$ increased		PKA reduced (Seyedi et al. 2005)		
	Ca^{2+} increased	Ca^{2+} increased	pERK1/2 increased (Lai et al. 2016)		
	cGMP increased L-type Ca^{2+} decreased	PKA increased	PLC inhibited (Lai et al. 2016)	PLC activated (Aldi et al. 2014)	
	NOS increased	GIRK increased	N- and L-type Ca^{2+} channels inhibited (Seyedi et al. 2005)		
	NO, NFκB increased	PP2A inhibited	Na$^+$ channel activation		
	PLA2 increased	PLC MAPK, increased	AT$_1$-R expression reduced (Hashikawa-Hobara et al. 2011)		

Receptor	H₁	H₂	H₃	H₄	Reference
cAMP-level	PLD, PKC increased	Moesin: more phosphorylated	NHE inhibition (Hashikawa-Hobara et al. 2011)		Del Tredici et al. 2013
	Phosphatidyl-3-kinase increased		PKG inhibited (Chan et al. 2012)	PKG inhibited (Chan et al. 2012)	
	MAPK increased		Ca^{2+} reduced (Sayedi et al. 2005)		

Here, practically relevant data for the four known histamine receptors (H_{1-4}) have been collected. In the second row the affinity of histamine to the four receptors is delineated. Of note, the H_4-receptor displays the highest and the H_2-histamine receptor the lowest affinity for histamine. Hence, receptors are expected to be activated, if all receptors were present in the same cell, in this order. The third and fourth rows present typical histamine receptor agonist and antagonist. Please note the for instance, dimaprit is agonist at both H_2-histamine receptors and H_4-histamine receptors, displaying poor selectivity. Histamine is of course agonist at all histamine receptor. Antagonists show better selectivity than agonists. Two antiarrhythmic agents (amiodarone and lorcainide) are unexpectedly antagonists at H_3-histamine receptors. Abbreviations: PKA, activity of cAMP-dependent protein kinase; PKG; activity of cGMP-dependent protein kinase Gs: stimulatory GTP-binding protein, Gi/o: inhibitory or other GTP-binding protein (can be inactivated by treatment with pertussis toxin), pERK1/2: phosphorylation state of extracellular signal regulated kinase 1 or 2, PLC: phospholipase C, PLA2, phospholipase A_2; PLD: phospholipase D; cAMP, level of 3´, 5´-cyclic adenosine monophosphate; cGMP, level of 3´, 5´-cyclic guanosine monophosphate; NOS, nitric oxide synthase, GIRK; activity of G protein-coupled inwardly-rectifying potassium channel, MAPK, activity of mitogen activated protein kinase; AT1-R, expression of angiotensin II receptor 1; PP2A, activity of the protein phosphatase 2A, Na^+: activity of sodium cation channel, NHE: activity of sodium cation and hydrogen exchanger, Ca^{2+} level of free Ca^{2+} in the cell, NO: concentration of nitric oxide, NFκB: expression of nuclear factor kappa-light-chain-enhancer of activated B-cells, IP_3: level of inositol-trisphosphate, PKC: activity of protein kinase C.

Mutations of HMT in patients with reduced and increased enzymatic activity of HMT are known (Jones and Kearns 2011, Yoshikawa et al. 2019): these mutations are expected to lead to higher or lower histamine levels in the heart, but these cardiac levels in mutation carriers have not yet been reported. HMT activity is reduced by some drugs (Table 3 in Yoshikawa et al. 2019). For instance, diphenhydramine, a H_1-histamine receptor antagonist (Table 4), in vitro and in vivo inhibits HMT (Adachi et al. 1992, 2011), which might raise histamine levels in the heart. Polymorphism of HMT exist which have 5-fold higher enzyme activities in patients (Jones and Kearns 2011). Cardiac consequences of these mutations have apparently not been studied. In addition, or alternatively some histamine can enter cells via the organic cation transporter-2 (OCT-2) or OCT-3 at least in some cells (Figure 1). It needs to be kept in mind that OCTs translocate histamine as a cation in both directions of cell membranes, be it in mast cells or cardiomyocytes (Ichikawa et al. 2010). It is unlikely that against a concentration gradient, histamine being at low concentrations in the plasma is transported via OCT-2 into the cardiomyocytes. At least in the heart, the concentration of histamine in the heart is unaltered (about 5 μM) by knocking out OCT-3 transporter questioning the role of this transporter (Ogasawara et al. 2006); however, more detailed work would be welcome. It seems more reasonable to hypothesize that histamine released locally from mast cells or other bloods cells very near the sarcolemma might use OCT-2 to enter cardiomyocytes. This hypothesis might not be valid in all regions of the human heart, because usually mast cell numbers are low in the ventricle and increase only in some diseased state. The MAO and DAO-inhibitor iproniazid, however, unexpectedly did not increase the formation of N-methyl-histamine plasma levels in psychiatric patients; only three patients were studied and more studies seem warranted (Lindell et al. 1960

5. Medical Use of Histamine

In some countries, histamine (given parenterally) is given in combination with other drugs for the treatment, for instance, of acute myeloid leukemia. In this case, histamine is thought to stimulate H_2-histamine receptors on leucocytes (Yang et al. 2011). This stimulation is intended to improve endogenous immune defense of the patient (Yang et al. 2011). This application of histamine is possibly accompanied with the known side of effects like tachycardia, bronchial constriction, reduction of blood pressure (Thoren et al. 2011, Yang und Perry 2011, Grauers Wiktorin et al. 2019). Impromidine, a selective agonist at H_2-histamine receptors has been used in the intensive care unit to treat acute heart failure (see below) with good mechanical improvement of the heart, but was abandoned due to reddening of the skin of patients and increased incidence of cardiac arrhythmias (Felix et al. 1995, see paragraph #15).

6. Histamine Receptors, Agonist and Antagonists

We now know that at least four histamine receptors exist (cellular expression reviewed in: Thangam et al. 2018) and all are found in the heart. They were chronologically labeled meaning that initially only one histamine receptor was assumed to exist and transmit all cardiac effects of histamine (Table 4). Later, data suggested that the same histamine receptor was responsible for gastric and cardiac responses are was different from the histamine receptor in the vascular smooth muscle and in the gut. Starting with a seminal paper (Black et al. 1972), compounds that stimulated and blocked preferentially cardiac inotropic effects in cavian preparations (H_2-histamine receptors involved) but not in cavian intestinal preparations (H_1-histamine receptors involved) became available. Several years later, H_1- and H_2-histamine receptors were cloned and could be used to study cardiac histamine receptors in much more molecular detail. About a decade later H_3-histamine receptors were cloned. DNA sequences that we now call H_4-histamine receptors were known to have sequences similar to the other known histamine receptors from the human genomic project, but their functional relevance was only later understood by studies on expressed H_4-histamine receptors in vitro.

H_3-histamine receptors and H_4-histamine receptors were initially thought to reside only in the central nervous system and in some blood cells. Only later when more selective agonists and selective H_3- and H_4-histamine receptor antagonists became available, progress in understanding the function of these receptors in the heart could be achieved. Based on these compounds (Table 4), H_3- and H_4-histamine receptors were thought to reside presynaptically on sympathetic nervous cells in the heart. Only recently, H_3-histamine receptors have been found in non-nerval structures in the heart: H_3-histamine receptors were convincingly detected in cardiac fibroblasts. H_4-histamine receptors apparently have not been reported to exist in non-neuronal cells in the heart, but we are not aware that any major effect has been put to detect H_3- and H_4-histamine receptors in cardiomyocytes especially human cardiomyocytes. Cardiac H_2-histamine receptors have recently been reviewed elsewhere and therefore will only get a cursory glance here (Neumann et al. 2021). With antibodies H_1- and H_2-histamine receptors are detected in cardiomyocytes of the atrium and ventricle of guinea pigs (Matsuda et al. 2004). Interestingly, these authors noted that the density of H_1- and H_2-histamine receptors in the sinus node cells and in atrioventricular-node cells were higher than in the surrounding atrial and possibly also the ventricular tissue (Matsuda et al. 2004). Hence, one can hypothesize that H_1- and H_2-histamine receptors are of special relevance in for the regulation and the conduction of the heartbeat. Hence, more efforts should be put into understanding their role better. It is conceivable that H_1-histamine receptors agonists or H_2-histamine receptors antagonists might be useful to treat atrial fibrillation. If one assumes the same to hold true in human heart, these receptors would easily explain why H_2-

histamine receptors agonists increase the beating rate (because they act stimulatory in the sinus node) and why H_2-histamine receptors agonist can hasten the signal propagation in the AV node. Moreover, this would explain why H_1-histamine receptors agonist reduce the beating rate of the heart and slow the AV conduction in human cardiac preparations (Genovese et al. 1988) and cavian cardiac preparations (Levi 1972, Levi and Kuye 1974, Levi et al. 1975). H_2-histamine receptor agonists have been used years ago in patients with end stage heart failure and improved their contractility. However, as far as we know a prospective randomized clinical study with the end point mortality in acute or chronic heart failure was never begun because at that time data came out that cAMP increasing agents like milrinone while improving heart failure killed the patient due to arrhythmias.

H_1-histamine receptor stimulation mediates in principle proinflammatory effects (Ichikawa et al. 2010). Part of this response is the increase in vascular permeability and results from the altered function of adhesion molecules in endothelial cells. H_2-histamine receptor stimulation leads to immune suppression, for instance, in macrophages (Ichikawa et al. 2010) which might be relevant in cardiac sepsis (paragraph #12) but also in ischemia and reperfusion damage (paragraph #10 and #11). The influence of histamine receptors on blood cells in cardiac function cannot obviously be studied when saline buffers are used in Langendorff-perfused heart or in atrial strips in the organ bath. However, very seldom nowadays blood is used for in vitro studies. Blood constituents can of course be studied for instance in experiments on myocardial infarction when the coronaries are ligated in living animals, which however is technically not trivial and involves permission from animal protection committees which are increasing difficult to get.

It has been known for some time that even in isolated atrium, histamine can be released, from intracardiac varicosities, by field stimulation (Li et al. 2004, 2006) and the release was impaired by H_3-histamine receptor stimulation (Li et al. 2006).

H_3-histamine receptors are expressed prejunctionally in sympathetic nerve endings and inhibit the release of noradrenaline and thus β-adrenergic effects (cavian atria: Endou et al. 1994, Luo et al. 1991, human atria: Imamura et al. 1995; canine heart: Mazenot et al. 1999a). After acute, short-lasting (about 10 min) cardiac ischemia when one reperfuses the heart, usually noradrenaline is released via exocytosis from the heart. This released noradrenaline is thought to be detrimental and might explain in part reperfusion injuries like cardiac arrhythmias because released noradrenaline activates β-adrenoceptors and increases cAMP content in the cardiomyocyte.

All cAMP increasing agents are known to increase the incidence of cardiac arrhythmias by altering Ca^{2+}-homeostasis in the heart and therefore, it is not surprising that released noradrenaline can induce arrhythmias. Histamine release from the heart during reperfusion after acute ischemia is thought to stimulate cardiac H_3-receptors. Indeed, a H_3-histamine receptor antagonist (thioperamide, Table 4 for synopsis) used during reperfusion, increased the release of noradrenaline during reperfusion of the heart (Imamura et al. 1994). During ischemia, histamine is thought to be released locally from cells in such numbers as to fully activate the H_3-histamine receptor so that stimulation of the receptor by an exogenous H_3-histamine receptor agonist cannot increase the noradrenaline release further (Immamura et al. 1994). Hence, one would predict that H_3-histamine receptor agonists would not have an additional beneficial effect in patients during coronary reperfusion in the catheter lab. In protracted ischemia (e.g., more than 20 min), noradrenaline is released from the heart by an additional process termed carrier mediated because the noradrenaline transporter (NET) is involved. Metaphorically, one could regard the NET as a revolving door that can transport noradrenaline into the cell or out of the cell. This revolving door can be put on hold by drugs like desimipramine or cocaine. Activation of NHE (the sodium hydrogen exchanger in outer cell membrane) is thought to facilitate the exit of noradrenaline from the cell by stimulation of NET. Conversely, if NHE is blocked, the outward transport of noradrenaline via the NET is blocked (cavian heart: Imamura et al. 1996, human heart: Hatta et al. 1997). Activation of H_3-histamine receptors under conditions of prolonged ischemia (more than 20 min) could reduce the (non-exocytotic) release of noradrenaline and this was accompanied by less arrhythmias (Imamura et al. 1996). This H_3-histamine receptor-mediated inhibition of noradrenaline release is species dependent, because this pathway is lacking in the rat heart (Mezenot et al, 1999b).

Sensory neurons in the heart (capsaicin-sensitive C-fibers) also contain functional H_3-histamine receptors. Calcitonin-related peptide (CGRP) can release histamine from cardiac mast cells and stimulate H_3-histamine receptors on C-fibers and this stimulation inhibits release of CGRP from these C-fibers in a similar fashion as H_3-histamine receptors inhibit noradrenaline release (Seyedi et al. 1999). In cardiac ischemia when protons accumulate and pH therefore falls, sensory C-fibers release more noradrenaline (Seyedi et al. 1999). Like many other G-protein coupled receptors, H_3-histamine receptors can form functional heterodimers with D_1-dopamine receptors in the brain (Moreno-Delgado et al. 2020). Whether such heterodimers are formed and will be functional in the heart needs to be elucidated but this is possible because D_1-dopamine receptors are present in the human heart (Ozono et al. 1997).

During reperfusion, application of drugs that reduce the release of noradrenaline could limit reperfusion injury (Chan et al. 2012). This assumption is supported by genetic studies: Isolated (Langendorff-perfused) hearts from mice with constitutive (i.e., not cardiac specific) KO of H_3-histamine receptors (Table 6) release more noradrenaline and show more decline in function and more cardiac arrhythmias upon reperfusion compared to wild type mice (Koyama et al. 2003a, b). The inhibitory action of H_3-histamine receptors on exocytosis of noradrenaline in cardiac ganglia was explained by two possibly synergistic pathways (Table 4): Firstly, H_3-histamine receptors inhibit via GTP-binding proteins the activity of neuronal adenylyl cyclase (Seyedi et al. 2005), cAMP levels fall and cAMP-dependent protein phosphorylation declines and thus the proteins involved in vesicular exocytosis remain inactive. Secondly, H_3-histamine receptors also activate a MAP kinase (Table 4) which finally ends in activation of a cyclo-oxygenase production of PGE2 and inhibition of Ca^{2+} entry into the nerve cell which will also impair release of noradrenaline from cardiac neuronal cells (Levi et al. 2007). Mast cells in the heart contain besides histamine also substantial amounts of renin (Silver et al. 2004). Renin initiate a cascade in the heart which finally forms angiotensin that can activate angiotensin receptors and these receptors again can increase the cardiac release of noradrenaline from neuronal cells. The release of renin from cardiac mast cells could be blocked by adding H_4-histamine receptor agonist to mast cells (Aldi et al. 2014). The putative cardioprotective role of H_4-histamine receptor activation is supported by the following observation. The detrimental effects of reperfusion were higher in isolated hearts treated with H_4-histamine receptor antagonists or hearts from H_4-histamine receptor KO mice than in wild type control hearts (Aldi et al. 2014).

Interestingly, H_3-histamine receptors and H_4-histamine receptors can also regulate vascular function in the heart (Figure 2). H_3-histamine receptor agonists induce endothelial dependent relaxation in the cerebral artery of the rabbit (Ea Kim et al. 1992). This was explained by H_3-histamine receptor mediated release of NO and PGE2, both of which are vasodilatory and are formed in the endothelial cells (Sun et al. 2010). H_3- and H_4-histamine receptor mRNA was found in cerebral endothelial cells and could lead there to production of NO (Karlstedt et al. 2013).

Furthermore, all four histamine receptors could be detected as mRNA and with antibodies in immunohistochemistry in human endothelial cells, specially, in human umbilical vein endothelial cells (HUVECs) and in human dermal microvascular endothelium (Adderley et al. 2015). One can extrapolate from these data to a similar situation in human cardiac coronary vessels but that has to be proven.

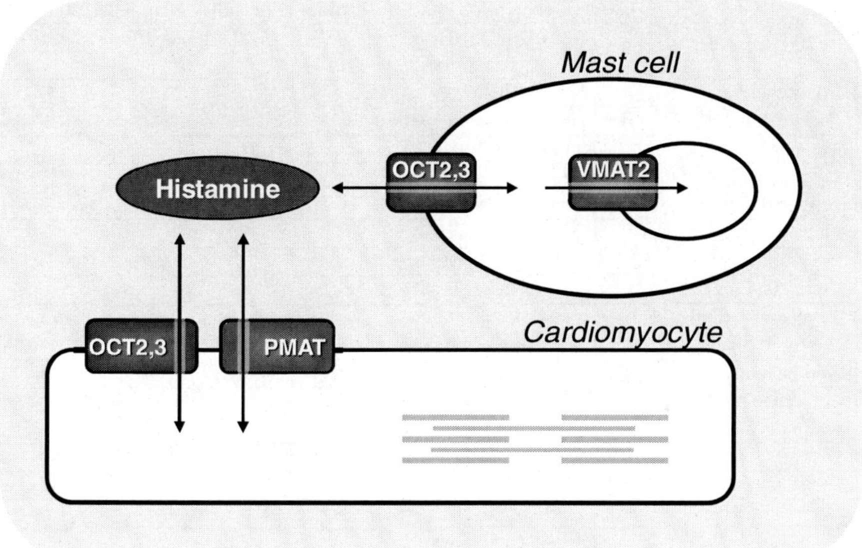

Figure 2. Uptake of histamine into cardiomyocytes.
Uptake of histamine into cardiomyocytes from the interstitium can be brought about by the plasma monoamine transporter (PMAT) and organic cation transporters (OCT) 2 or OCT 3. Via OCT 2 or 3, histamine could enter and leave the mast cell. Within mast cells, vesicular monoamine transporter 2 (VMAT2) can transport histamine from the cytosol into the vesicles of the mast cells. These transporters can be blocked by organic molecules (Table 5).

In myofibroblasts from adult rat hearts, H_3-histamine receptors were detected with an H_3-histamine receptor antibody; however, control experiments for the specificity of the H_3-histamine receptor antibody, a notorious problem in G-protein coupled receptors (Seifert et al. 2013) was apparently not performed, likewise mRNA data were missing.

However, the authors could pharmacologically detect the function of these H_3-histamine receptors: Imetit stimulated collagen deposition in these myofibroblasts in culture. The effect was specific because a H_3-histamine receptor antagonist, was ineffective under these conditions to block histamine induce collagen production (Piera et al. 2019) their stimulation in mouse heart

H_3-histamine receptor mRNA expression was found and confirmed by mRNA sequencing of one isoform (McCaffrey et al. 2020).

Table 5. Drugs or diseases or interventions known to release histamine into the plasma

Drugs	
Vancomycin	Goodman and Gilman 13.edition, Polk 1991, Gergs et al. 2021
Morphine (and derivates)	Goodman and Gilman 13. edition, Meyler´s side effects of drugs 15. Edition, Gergs et al. 2021
Doxorubicin	rabbit: Bristow et al. 1981
Tachycardia	Wolff and Levi 1986
Ketamine	Costa-Farré et al. 2005, Gergs et al. 2021
Calcitonin Gene-Related Peptide (CGRP)	Mast cells, guinea pig heart: Imamura et al. 1996
Inhalation narcosis	Meyer-Burgdorff et al. 1976
Neurotensin	Gi-mediated: Mousli et al. 1990
Compound 48/80	Gi-mediated: Mousli et al. 1990
Tubocurarin (and other Curare-derivatives	Goodman and Gilman 13. edition, Meyler´s side effects of drugs 15 edition, guinea pig: Giotti et al. 1966
Adriamycin	Rat heart: Decorti et al. 1997
Histamine producing tumors	Uccella et al. 2006
Diseases	
LPS-mediated: sepsis	Oguri et al. 2003
Bacteria-mediated sepsis	Carlos et al. 2013, Matsuda et al. 2002
Decreased DAO activity by drugs	Maintz and Novak 2007
Decreased DAO activity by food ingredients	Maintz and Novak 2007
Urticaria pigmentosa	Goodman and Gilman 13.edition, Shaffer et al. 2006, Rohr et al. 2005
Rheumatoid arthritis	Tetlow and Woolley 2005
Systemic mastocytosis	Goodman and Gilman 13 .edition Shaffer et al. 2006, Rohr et al. 2005, Andersen et al. 2012
Myeloid leukemia	Goodman and Gilman 13. edition; Sperr et al. 2002
Inflammation	Jutel 2009
Graft versus host reactions	Jutel 2009
Transplantation	Inoue et al. 2007
Arteriosclerosis	Gill et al. 1989
Anaphylaxis	Rutkowski et al. 2012
Myocardial infarction in patients	Luo et al. 2013

Interventions	
Stress (cage restraint)	Mouse hearts : Huang et al. 2002
Extracorporeal circulation	Meyer-Burgdorff et al. 1976

It might be of interest, which drugs a patient has taken, or which diseases the patient suffers from because this might interfere with histamine studies. On the other hand, one can argue that the untoward cardiac effects of histamine might be brought about or might be at least potentiated by the drugs, interventions and diseases listed in Table 13. There are many drugs known to release histamine and lead to local (for instance cutaneous, leading to reddish colors of the skin) or systemically high concentrations of histamine in organs or the serum of patients. One can assume that these drugs or diseases might increase also cardiac concentrations of histamine, though that has seldom been reported. Caution again is warranted: while several drugs can release histamine from mast cells in the skin this is not necessarily the case in cardiac mast cells or is often even not yet known. Moreover, inhibition of DAO means inhibition of diamine oxidase in the gut or in the whole body: this inhibition will increase the bioavailability of histamine or increase its concentration in the blood in directly in the heart.

Table 6. Genetic models in cardiac histamine research

Protein	Reference	Model		Inhibitors drugs
	Inoue et al. 1996	Constitutive KO		See Table 1
H_2-histamine receptors	Gergs et al. 2019	Cardiac specific overexpression		
H_2-histamine receptors	Kobayashi et al. 2000, Fukushima et al. 2003		Constitutive KO	See Table 1
H_3-histamine receptors	Toyota et al. 2002, Takahashi et al. 2002		Constitutive KO	See Table 1
H_4-histamine receptors	Hofstra et al. 2003		Constitutive KO	See Table 1
HDC	Othsu et al. 2001	Histidine decarboxylase is pace making enzyme	Constitutive KO	NSD-1055, Quinacrine, α-fluoromethyl-histidine Levine et al. 1965, Duggan et al. 1984
HDC	Walker et al. 2013	Tissue specific localization of HDC	Cre-mouse X Reporter mouse	
HDC	Yamada et al. 2020		HDC-floxed mouse	
Histamine N-Methyl-transferase	Yoshikawa et al. 2019		Constitutive KO	Quinacrine, SKF 91488, Yohikawa et al. 2013, Sattler et al. 1985

Table 6. (Continued)

Protein	Reference	Model		Inhibitors drugs
MAO-A	Cases et al. 1995		Constitutive KO	Clorgyline Waldmeier et al. 1977
MAO-A OE	Kaludercic et al. 2010, Villeneuve et al. 2013		Overexpression	
MAO-B	Grimsby et al. 1997		Constitutive KO	Pargyline, selegiline Waldmeier et al. 1977
Diaminoxidase	Stolen et al. 2005		Constitutive KO	Dihydralazine, aminoguanidine, chloroquine,
				tubocurarin, ethanol (Sattler et al. 1985), Rhodanine (Dai 1987)
Alcohol dehydrogenase	Oyama et al. 2005	Only heterozygous survive	Constitutive KO	Fomepizol (4-methylpyrazole), disulfiram (Papp et al. 1984, Moore and Drury 1951)
Xanthinoxidase	Ohtsubo et al. 2004		Constitutive KO	Allopurinol Elion et al. 1966
Dopa-Decarboxylase	Zhang et al. 2011		Floxed mice	Benserazide, NSD 1015, Del Valle and Gantz 1997, Levine et al. 1965
Imidazole acetate-phosphoribosyl-diphosphate-ligase	Not available?			Sodium salicylate Moss et al. 1976
OCT2	Gründemann 1998 b	Constitutive KO	See Table 2	Duan and Wang 2010, Soetanto et al. 2019
OCT3	Zwart et a. 2001	Constitutive KO	See Table 2	Duan and Wang 2010, Soetanto et al. 2019

Protein	Reference	Model		Inhibitors drugs
VMAT2	Takahashi et al. 2013	Constitutive KO	See Table 2	Travis et al. 2000, Soetanto et al. 2019
PMAT	Duan and Wang 2010	Constitutive KO	See Table 2	Soetanto et al. 2019

Here, knock out mice or floxed mice or overexpression mice for the study of histamine and its receptors in the heart are presented. Instead of using a genetically engineered mouse, it is often a useful first step to display specificity of effects. Especially, when studying effects in humans it might be helpful before trying a genetic approach, to test small organic molecules having displayed here as more or less specific inhibitor of enzyme activity. Sometimes it is of interest to study a function solely in heart and one does not want to alter the biochemistry in other organs because this may complicate the identification of special pathways. Then a genetic approach with floxed mice and heart cell specific reporter mice might be considered.

The levels of H_3-histamine receptors mRNA expression were similar in cardiac samples from control mice and samples from wild type mice treated with angiotensin II (as a stressor given parenterally for seven days): in contrast, protein levels for H_3-histamine receptors were only detected (using Western blotting) in angiotensin II treated hearts, but not in untreated hearts (McCaffrey et al. 2020). Further analysis revealed that the signal for H_3-histamine receptors was derived from fibroblasts in the mouse heart. Activation of H_3-histamine receptors with imetit reduced the angiotensin II-induced fibrosis in mice while blocking H_3-histamine receptors was without effect (McCaffrey et al. 2020). These data convincingly show that H_3-histamine receptors occur not only on nerve cells but also on other cell types in the heart and can be of (patho)physiological relevance. One wonders if under stressful conditions protein expression and thus altered function of H_3-histamine receptors (and H_4-histamine receptors) in cardiomyocytes might occur.

It is not without precedence that the various cell types of an organ contain cell specific expression of the histamine receptors: such is the case in the kidney where the glomeruli contain only H_1-histamine and H_2-histamine receptors and the H_3-histamine receptor is confined to the collecting duct and the H_4-histamine receptor to the ascending limb of the loop of Henle (Grange et al. 2020): a similar cell specific expression of histamine receptors is conceivable in the heart, but needs to be proven.

7. Effects of Histamine on Force of Contraction and Beating Rate

The effects of histamine on force and beating rate show region specific- and species- dependent effects. In human atrial preparations, H_2-histamine receptors lead to an increase in force of contraction (Ginsburg et al. 1980). Contradictory reports exists, surprisingly, on the role of H_1-histamine receptors: H_1-histamine receptors stimulation was reported lead to a reduction in force of contraction in isolated human atrial preparations (Genovese et al. 1988) or an increase in force of contraction in human atrial preparations (Sanders et al. 1996). The reason(s) for this discrepancies are not readily apparent, as both labs are very experienced in the field. Conceivably, co-medication or patient co-morbidities might play a role, but this issue should be addressed anew. In the sinus node and the atrioventricular node, H_2-histamine receptors increase the heart rate and the conduction and these effects were antagonized by H_1-histamine receptor stimulation (Genovese et al. 1988, Zerkowski et al. 1993, Ginsburg et al. 1980). In ventricular human preparations, histamine seems to augment force of contraction via H_2-histamine receptors (Ginsburg et al. 1980; Bristow et al. 1982a). However, also H_1-histamine receptors exist in the human ventricle (biochemically detected in Northern and Western blots: Matsuda et al. 2004) and have been reported to decrease force of contraction in isolated ventricular muscle strips (Du et al. 1993). More efforts using more selective and potent agonists in the human heart might be worthwhile. Pigs often are sometimes used in circulation research because the porcine heart size is similar to human hearts. Positive inotropic effects via H_2-histamine receptors are noted in the porcine atrium and but H_1-histamine receptors mediate a reduction in force of contraction in porcine ventricles (Du et al. 1993). Thus, porcine ventricle is a poor model of the human heart as concerns histamine receptor function. Also dogs have been studied because they have a coronary system in many ways similar to humans. While the H_2-histamine receptor mediated the positive inotropic effect of histamine in the canine ventricle, the positive inotropic effect in the canine atrium are solely H_1-histamine receptor mediated and thus do not resemble human atrium in this regard (Chiba 1976, Endoh 1979). In both, rabbit atrium and ventricle, H_2-histamine receptors mediate a small positive inotropic effect via cAMP, but the H_1-histamine receptor mediated the main component of the positive inotropic effects (Hattori et al. 1988, 1990). In cavian left atrium, only H_1-receptors mediate a positive inotropic effect and only H_1-histamine receptors mediate chronotropic effects in the cavian right atrium. However, in the ventricle of guinea pigs, both H_1- and H_2-histamine receptors mediated positive inotropic effects (Verma and McNeill 1977, Macleod et al. 1986, Sakuma et al. 1988b). Finally, it needs to be mentioned that data in rat (Bartlet 1963, Laher and McNeil 1980a), feline hearts (Laher and McNeil 1980c) and mice (Gergs et al. 2019, Gergs et al. 2020) indicate that these animals do not exhibit functional histamine receptors but histamine in these species releases noradrenaline which then increases force of contraction and heart rate by acting on β-adrenoceptors.

8. Electrophysiological Effects

Histamine can increase currents through L-type Ca^{2+} channels and increased delayed outward potassium currents (I_K) in isolated cavian ventricular cardiomyocytes (Hescheler et al. 1987). These effects are in all likelihood mediated by an increase in cAMP-levels in the cardiomyocyte and a subsequent increase in the activity of the cAMP-dependent protein kinase and based on use of specific agonists like dimaprit and antagonists like cimetidine are mediated by H_2-histamine receptors (Table 4). Likewise, the effects of histamine on the potassium currents were cimetidine-sensitive and hence were also regarded as H_2-histamine receptor-mediated in isolated cavian ventricular cardiomyocytes (Yazawa and Abiko 1993, Tanaka et al. 1991). The histamine-induced increase in potassium currents in cavian ventricular cardiomyocytes was reduced by additionally applied carbachol (a derivative of acetylcholine); which was interpreted as evidence of an antagonism at the adenylyl cyclase level between effects of histamine on H_2-histamine receptors and carbachol on M_2-muscarinic receptors (Tanaka et al. 1991). At certain concentrations, histamine could also increase in potassium currents which would shorten the duration of action potentials in these cells and this shortening of the action potential duration was predicted to produce arrhythmias in patients (Yazawa and Abiko 1993) and would also reduce the force of contraction as less time would be available for trigger Ca^{2+} to enter the cardiomyocytes. In addition, histamine can increase currents through chloride currents in cavian ventricular cardiomyocytes which might lead to impaired conduction and possibly might also lead to arrhythmias (Harvey and Hume 1989). There are regional differences in the electrophysiological effects of histamine which are in line with the regional differences in the positive inotropic effects of histamine: in cavian left atrial cardiomyocytes, H_1-histamine receptors mediated an increase in intracellular Ca^{2+} levels which was not accompanied by a direct activation of L-type Ca^{2+} channels (Yoshimoto et al. 1998), but because H_1-histamine receptor stimulation prolongs the open state of a potassium channel: this prolongs the duration of the action potential and therefore more time is available for Ca^{2+} to enter the cells, probably through the L-type Ca^{2+} channel current (Yoshimoto et al. 1998, Amerini et al. 1982, Borchard and Hafner, 1986a,b, Hattori et al. 1988a). In the sinus node of rabbits, histamine via H_2-histamine receptors could increase the hyperpolarization activated current (HCN or I_f-current), the current through L-type Ca^{2+} channel and potassium currents, which were accompanied by an increase in beating rate and a reduction of action potential duration (APD): these effects were antagonized by additionally applied acetylcholine which often induced arrhythmias (Satoh 1993). The effects are also usually explained by an acetylcholine-mediated inhibition of histamine stimulated activity of adenylyl cyclase in sinus node cells. In human multicellular cardiac preparations (papillary muscle strips from the left ventricle of patients with mitral valve lesions), histamine (and dimaprit) increased the duration of the action potential, increased the height and duration of the plateau phase of the action potential (Eckel et al. 1982) which, in principle, could lead to arrhythmias in patients. In spontaneously contracting right atrial muscle strips (obtained during cardiac surgery) from patients, histamine increased the beating rate, the maximum diastolic potential, the amplitude of the action potential and automaticity; these effects were verapamil-sensitive and thus probably driven by influx of Ca^{2+} via the L-type Ca^{2+} channels (Levi et al. 1981). Histamine was less potent in these experiments on isolated atrial preparations than epinephrine (=adrenaline) (Levi et al. 1981): this could mean that the H_2-histamine receptor density on cardiomyocytes (which is not known, only on cardiac homogenates: Matsuda et al. 2004), is lower than the density of β-adrenoceptors or that they couple less effectively to intracellular messengers. Measurements of cytosolic Ca^{2+} in cardiomyocytes would clarify these open questions. In some human right atrial samples, histamine induced delayed afterdepolarizations and triggered activity which was blocked by cimetidine but not by propranolol and thus the human (albeit in vitro) arrhythmias (for more details see below) were convincingly regarded as H_2-histamine receptor mediated (Levi et al. 1981).

9. Effects on Vessels

Effects on coronary arteries (Figure 2; Table 2): Histamine can lead to vasodilatation due to H_2-histamine receptor and/or H_1-histamine receptor mediated vasodilatation (perfused cavian heart: Levi and Kuye 1974) or to H_1-histamine receptor mediated vasoconstriction (summarized in Table 2). These effects are different not only in different species but in different regions of the mammalian body as well (Table 2). In humans, these effects are even disease-dependent. Moreover, histamine can elicit both vasodilatation and vasoconstriction in the very same vessel in a concentration- and time-dependent fashion. Nowadays a floxed H_2-histamine receptor mouse is available (Meng et al. 2021) and using these mice is should be possible to knock out the H_2-histamine receptor in a region- and tissue-specific fashion in mice at will. Such data would be valuable. In old studies, histamine led to contraction in isolated mouse thoracic aortae pre-contracted with 0.1 µM norepinephrine (Van de Voorde and Leusen 1982; mouse strain not reported). In isolated aortae of wild type mice (CD1-strain) lower concentrations of histamine induced vasorelaxation whereas at higher concentrations of histamine led to vasoconstriction but in other WT strains (black six) histamine only led to vasoconstriction (Schlegel et al. 2015). At least in CD1 WT mice injection of histamine in the peritoneum led to vasoconstriction as measured by Doppler ultrasound measurements (Schlegel et al. 2015).

In human umbilical vascular endothelial cells (HUVEC), histamine does not increase cAMP-levels but increases the phosphorylation state of myosin light chain either by activation of a myosin light chain kinase or an inhibition of myosin light chain phosphatase and increases subsequently the permeability of endothelial cell layers (Moy et al. 1993). At least in corneal endothelial cells in culture, the mRNA and the protein for H_1-histamine receptors could be measured in these endothelial cells and their activation of a myosin light chain kinase but also histamine also inhibited a myosin light chain phosphatase (Srinivas et al. 2006). The inhibition of this phosphatase in endothelial cells might result from an enhanced PKC-induced phosphorylation of a protein that when phosphorylated acts as a phosphatase inhibitor (PKC-potentiated inhibitory protein of 17 kDa=CPI-17: Kolosova et al. 2004, Eto et al. 2001). Phosphorylated CPI-17 inhibits the catalytic subunit of PP1δ, which can bind to a so called myosin phosphatase targeting subunit 1 (MYPT1, reviewed: Herzig and Neumann 2000, Liu 2021). This MYPT1 in endothelial cells can be phosphorylated an inactivated by a Rho kinase and phosphorylated MYPT1 inactivates PP1 δ, thus inhibits myosin light chain phosphatase activity in endothelial cells and therefore can lead to an increased phosphorylation state and therefore probably increased endothelial cellular permeability (review: Kamm and Stull 2001). Alternatively, or additionally, H_1-histamine receptor stimulation in endothelial cells will increase intracellular free Ca^{2+}; this will activate a myosin light chain kinase again leading to an increase in the phosphorylation state of myosin light chains review (Kamm and Stull 2001). H_1-histamine receptor stimulation in smooth muscle cells leads to vasoconstriction probably due to the known increase histamine induces in myosin light chain phosphorylation (tracheal muscle: Kamm et al. 1989, swine carotid artery: van Riper et al. 1995). In isolated coronary arteries of swine, potassium induced a vasoconstriction in the organ bath; thereafter cumulatively, histamine was applied and this led to further vasoconstriction (Yamamoto et al. 1987). This vasoconstriction was slightly attenuated by removal of the endothelium (Yamamoto et al. 1987): this strongly suggests that vasodilation due to histamine receptors (H_1-histamine receptors and H_2-histamine receptors) on endothelial cells is only responsible for fine tuning of histamine-induced vasoconstriction (due to H_1-histamine receptors on smooth muscle cells). It is believed that H_1-histamine receptors on smooth muscle cells in the coronary arteries lead to myosin light chain phosphorylation via the mechanism mentioned above for endothelial cells. In pulmonary arterial rings from rats, dimaprit induced at most 50% relaxation, whereas isoproterenol (1 µM) induced complete relaxation (after pre-contraction with potassium cations): this was regarded as evidence for a H_2-histamine receptor mediated effect (Fullerton et al. 1996). In human endothelial cells, histamine led to increased production of NO directly measured (Lantoine et al. 1998). This might be due to a H_2-histamine receptor mediated increase in cAMP which will activate PKA and PKA can phosphorylate and activate endothelial nitric oxide synthase (eNOS) increasing the enzymatic activity of eNOS and thus NO production in the smooth muscle cell (Mount et al. 2007). Enhanced NO leads to increased activity of guanylyl cyclase in the smooth muscle cell, increased levels of cGMP, reduced Ca^{2+} levels and finally relaxation (review: Golshiri et al. 2020). Segments from porcine aorta, responded to histamine with enhanced measurable production of NO which was gone when endothelial cells were mechanically removed and was cimetidine sensitive and not accompanied by an increase in cellular free Ca^{2+} (Kishi et al. 1998). In these segments, histamine induced contractions which were increased by addition of cimetidine, suggesting that H_2-histamine receptor-mediated relaxation had taken place which was overcome by H_1-histamine receptor-mediated vasoconstriction (Kishi et al. 1998). H_1-histamine receptor stimulation in HUVEC leads via a receptor operated channel to an influx of extracellular Ca^{2+} which bind to calmodulin and this complex than activated a NO synthase thus elevating cellular NO production and NO content and NO can act in endothelial cells or diffuse to other cells or cell types (Lantoine et al. 1998).

Hence, the vascular effects of histamine are not trivial and if one interpreted experiments in living mice one would have to be very careful in order to translate these findings properly to the clinic. The situation in the human coronaries is the most relevant, best studied by far, but not without apparent contradictions, perhaps due to gender, age of patients, preexisting conditions, surgical procedures, drug treatment before surgery or at the time of surgery, the time between dissection in the theatre and the organ bath experiments; in some cases, post mortem coronary samples were used suggesting possible death of cells in coronary arteries. There seems to be one constant finding: both vasoconstriction and vasodilatation after histamine addition to strips of human coronary arteries in the organ bath can be observed. In left and right coronary arteries from heart transplant recipients, histamine exerted vasoconstriction via H_1-histamine receptors and vasodilation via H_2-histamine-receptors (Ginsburg et al. 1980, Toda 1983). Histamine was more potent in proximal than in distal segments of human epicardial coronary arteries (Ginsburg et al. 1984). Removal of the endothelium led to potentiation of the vasoconstrictor effect of histamine (Toda 1987). Individual differences appeared: 60% of human coronaries reacted with vasoconstriction and 40% with vasodilation (Toda 1987); this was suggested to result from different densities of mast cells in patients: mast cells contain high concentrations of histamine which can be released (Okumura et al. 1991). In the presence of intact endothelium, the vasodilatory effect of histamine was accompanied by and probably caused by an increase of 3',5'-cyclic guanosine monophosphate (cGMP) in the human coronary strips (Toda and Okamura 1989). The interpretation was: there are both, H_1- and H_2-histamine receptors in coronary smooth muscle cells and only H_1-histamine receptors in endothelial cells (Toda and Okamura 1989). In contrast to this view, in animal studies it turned out that H_2-histamine receptors can also reside in endothelial cells and there they can increase cAMP-levels (bovine aortic endothelial cells: Hekimian et al. 1992) which might via phosphorylate and therefore activate a NO synthase. This NO diffuses into the neighboring smooth muscle cells. In this this way, H_2-histamine receptors on endothelial cells can lead to vasodilatation (and in bovine aortic endothelial cells reduced permeability for albumin: Hekimian et al. 1992). At least using mice with endothelial specific knock out of H_2-histamine receptors, it has been convincingly shown that H_2-histamine receptors are biochemically present on endothelial cells (Meng et al. 2021): detailed functional studies in this model are not yet available in the literature.

In vivo, in humans, if cimetidine is given to block H_2-histamine receptors, peripheral infusion of histamine in probands (without coronary heart disease) decreased the coronary resistance.

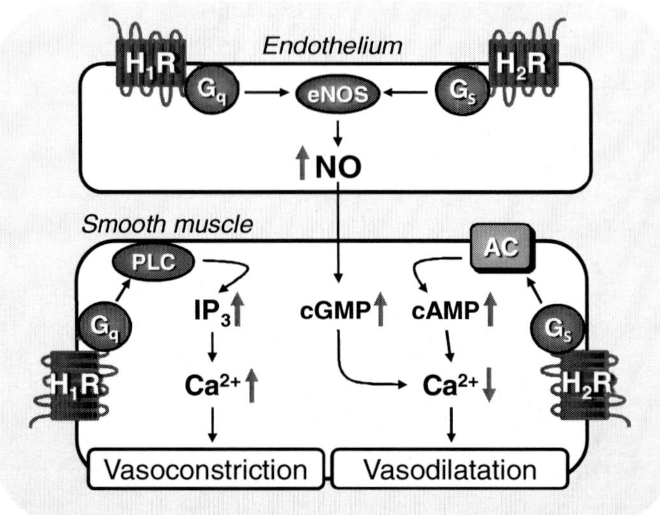

Figure 3. Histamine receptors in peripheral blood vessels. In the endothelium, both H_1-histamine receptors (H_1R) and H_2-histamine receptors (H_2R) are expressed and both can activate endothelial nitric oxide synthase (eNOS) which forms NO. This NO diffuses into surrounding smooth muscle cells and there activates guanylyl cyclases which increases cGMP-levels. Produced cGMP may activate cGMP-dependent protein phosphorylation or may inhibit phosphodiesterase activity increase cAMP-levels and activate cAMP-dependent phosphorylation. Finally, Ca^{2+} content in the smooth muscle is reduced and this leads to vasodilation. On the other hand, H_2R exist on smooth muscle cells and they increase cAMP-content, which via protein phosphorylation reduces Ca^{2+}-levels and thereby also lead to vasodilatation. The stimulation of H_1R on smooth muscle cells can increase inositol-tri-phosphate-(IP_3) content, IP_3 releases Ca^{2+} and therefore free Ca^{2+} is increased and this may lead to vasoconstriction. Alternatively, H_1R-stimulation may also activate myosin light chain kinases or may inhibit myosin light chain phosphatases in smooth muscle cells (see Figure 7). Because some uncertainties exist, we have not depicted here that H_3-histamine receptors and H_4-histamine receptors are likewise present in human endothelial cells. H_3-histamine receptor and/or H_4-histamine receptor stimulation may lead to production of vasodilatory prostaglandins in endothelial cells (Figure 6, 7) that diffuse to smooth muscle cells in the vicinity and thus lead to vasodilatation (modified from Cianchi et al. 2005).

This was regarded as evidence that in vivo H_1-histamine receptors mediate vasodilatation (Vigorito et al. 1986a, 1987). In the coronary arteries (as in the heart muscle cells), histamine can be formed locally or histamine can enter the coronaries with the blood stream (Keitoku 1990). Further clarity came from experiments where not histamine (which acts in all H_1-, H_2-, H_3-, H_4-histamine receptors) but the H_2-histamine agonist impromidine was used in patients and led to a decline in blood pressure which was cimetidine-sensitive and can be regarded as further evidence that H_2-histamine receptors are present in the periphery and their stimulation can lead to vascular dilatation in healthy persons (Boyce 1982).

10. Ischemia

It is well established and has been noted in various animal models by independent groups that after cardiac ischemia during reperfusion high concentrations of histamine leave the heart (awake dog with coronary ligation: Masini et al. 1985; guinea pig: Levi et al. 1985; rat: Valen et al.1994a; mouse: He et al. 2012; human after cardioplegic arrest: Valen et al. 1994b). As mentioned above, if one reduces the release of noradrenaline in ischemia, less damage like arrhythmias is caused by ischemia (Hatta et al. 1997). H_3- and H_4-histamine receptors might act in a beneficial way, because they can impair the release of noradrenaline from neuronal structures also in the human heart (Imamura et al. 1995). The H_3-histamine receptor was regarded as non-activated under physiological conditions (review: Levi and Smith 2000). However, in reperfusion after 10 min ischemia in isolated perfused cavian hearts the H_3-histamine receptor antagonist thioperamide could increase the amount of noradrenaline released from the heart as measured in the eluate, presumably because the normal H_3-histamine receptor mediated inhibition of noradrenaline release was reversed (Imamura et al. 1994). This reduction in noradrenaline release is also thought to reduce the incidence of reperfusion arrhythmias (Imamura et al. 1996). There seems to be a protective feedback in the heart via released histamine. Ischemia alters the mitochondrial metabolism in the heart: more acetaldehyde is formed and released from cardiac mitochondria because oxidation is impaired. This acetaldehyde and possible free radicals can release renin from mast cells residing in cardiac tissue. Renin, a protease, finally leads to the generation of angiotensin II, which acts on (Figure 3) its receptors in cardiac ganglia. The activity of NHE is thereby increased and this leads to release of noradrenaline from the cardiac ganglia and stimulation of cardiac β-adrenoceptors on cardiomyocytes and thus to cAMP increases altered Ca^{2+} homeostasis, exit of Ca^{2+} from the cell via the electrogenic Ca^{2+} exchanger, thereby to premature depolarization and finally to cardiac arrhythmias. Fortunately, not only renin but also histamine is released from mast cells at the same time. This released histamine can in an autocrine or paracrine fashion stimulate mast cell H_4-histamine receptors to stop the release of renin (Mackins et al., 2006, Aldi et al. 2014). Interestingly,

H_2-histamine receptors seem to exert a protective role in the cardiac atrium against hypoxia and a detrimental role in ischemia in the left ventricle (Gergs et al. 2020a).

11. Myocardial Infarction

In mice (Chen et al. 2017), in dogs (Masini et al. 1985) and in patients (Chen et al. 2017, Luo et al. 2013, Zdravkovic et al. 2011), myocardial infarction was accompanied by increased plasma levels of histamine. But also in patients with angina pectoris, elevated plasma histamine levels were reported (Zdravkovic et al. 2011). This increase in histamine has been suggested to be mediated by action of free radicals on mast cells in the heart and from these mast cells histamine is released and acts directly on surrounding cardiomyocytes or enters the blood stream and leaves the heart (Pierpaoli et al. 2003). Others presented data that after myocardial infarction, induction of HDC levels in immune cells of the heart occurs and this might explain detrimental effects of histamine in myocardial infarction (Chen et al. 2017). After occlusion and reperfusion, histamine release has been described for instance in the isolated perfused cavian heart (Genovese et al. 1988) and histamine might also be released from mast cells in the heart (Masini et al. 1991). In a similar way, in ischemia, histamine is released from mast cells in human hearts (Reid et al. 2011). A protective role of histamine in infarction has also been suggested: low concentrations of histamine can lead via H_2-histamine receptor to vasodilation of coronary arteries in experimental animals. After cardiac ischemia and reperfusion arrhythmias occurred in WT mouse hearts; the incidence of arrhythmias was smaller in mice lacking HDC than in WT mice, and was reduced by the H_2-histamine receptor antagonist famotidine, implying a causative role of histamine in these arrhythmias (He et al. 2012). In living mice where ischemia and reperfusion was surgically induced, famotidine given in WT mice or use of H_2-histamine receptor KO mice exhibited less severe cardiac necrosis than in untreated WT mice (Luo et al. 2013). Also in living dogs, H_2-histamine receptor blockers reduced infarct size, when infarct was surgically induced (Asanuma et al. 2006).

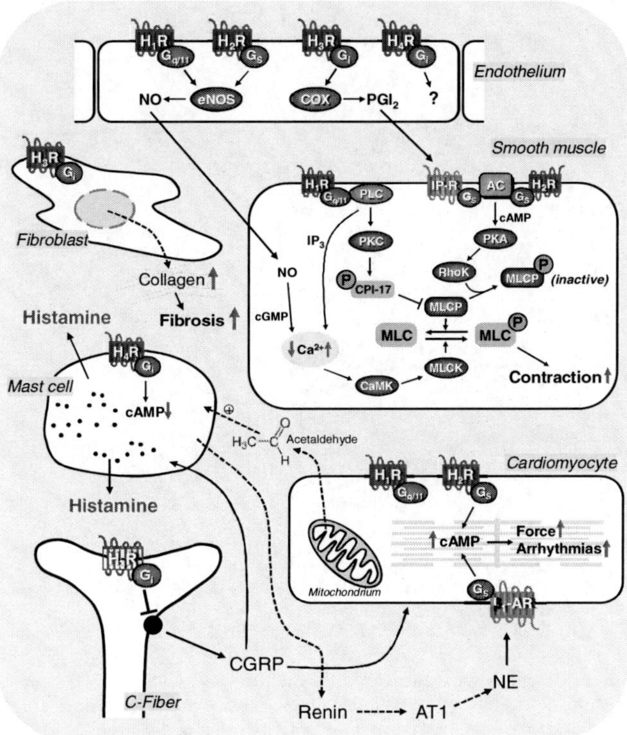

Figure 4. Synopsis of histamine and histamine receptors in the heart. Endothelial cells contain all four types of histamine receptors. H_1- and H_2-histamine receptor stimulation leads via GTP-binding proteins eventually to phosphorylation and thereby to activation of endothelial nitric oxide synthase (eNOS) and thus to production of NO. This NO diffuses into neighboring smooth muscle where soluble guanylyl cyclase is stimulated and produces cGMP. This activates cGMP-dependent kinases which finally phosphorylates proteins that initiate a decline in cellular Ca^{2+} that leads to muscle relaxation. H_3-histamine receptors in endothelial cells are thought to stimulate a cyclo-oxygenase (COX) that will form prostaglandin I_2 that likewise diffuses into smooth muscle cells increases there cAMP and via cAMP dependent protein kinase leads to decline in cellular Ca^{2+} and relaxation (see Figure 7). The role of the endothelial H_4-histamine receptor is unclear. H_1-histamine receptor stimulation on smooth muscle cells (Figure 7 for details) lead via PLC to activation of PKC which leads to an increase in Ca^{2+}. This Ca^{2+} binds to calmodulin that activates a myosin light chain kinase (MLCK). The MLCK phosphorylates myosin light chains (MLC) and this leads to muscle contraction. This process is amplified because PLC also activates via PKC the CPI-17. This protein inhibits myosin light chain phosphatase and this also increases the phosphorylation state of MLC and thus contributes to contraction. The stimulation of H_3 histamine receptors on fibroblasts can lead to fibrosis. H_2-histamine receptor stimulation in cardiomyocytes leads to a cAMP-increase and subsequent increase in contractility. The role of the H_1-histamine receptor on cardiomyocytes is controversial. Under hypoxic conditions, cardiac myocytes produce in the mitochondria acetaldehyde which releases histamine from mast cells but also proteases like renin. Renin produces finally angiotensin II, which releases noradrenaline from neuronal cells and this can act on β-adrenoceptors on cardiomyocytes to increase cAMP content which can lead to cardiac arrhythmias. Histamine released from mast cells can stimulate H_3-histamine receptors on neuronal C-fibers. This will inhibit the release of calcitonin-gene related peptide (CGRP) which otherwise could diffuse to cardiomyocytes and increase cardiac contractility. The release of renin and histamine stimulated by acetaldehyde from mast cells is inhibited by H_4-receptor stimulation (Modified from Imamura et al. 1996b, Srinivas et al. 1996, Hattori et al. 1996, Panula et al. 2015, Aldi et al. 2014).

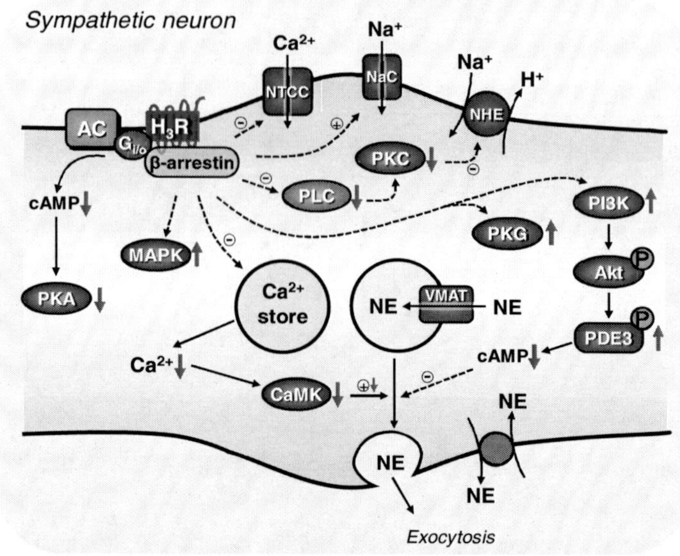

Figure 5. Signal transduction of H₃-histamine receptors in the heart.
Heptahelical H₃-histamine receptors in sympathetic ganglions or other cell types can inhibit the activity of cardiac adenylyl cyclases (AC) via pertussis-sensitive GTP- binding proteins ($G_{i/o}$). This leads to a fall in cAMP content and subsequent less activity of cAMP-dependent protein kinases (PKA) which results in less phosphorylation and thus less activity of substrates for PKA. Substrates include the neuronal Ca^{2+} channel (NTCC). Less activity of NTCC leads to less Ca^{2+} entering the cell and thus less free Ca^{2+} in the cell. An increase in free Ca^{2+} would mean that Ca^{2+} binds to calmodulin and subsequent activation of a Ca^{2+}/calmodulin-dependent protein kinase (CaMK) and this kinase phosphorylates and activates proteins that lead to the exocytosis of noradrenaline (NE) which then leaves the cell and increases in the interstitium. This NE may enter again the cell via the bidirectional NE-transporting protein (NET). NE taken up into the cell may get degraded by monoamine oxidases in the mitochondria (not shown), may remain for some time in the cytosol or NE may be actively transported against a gradient into storage vesicles in the cell by a transporting enzyme called vesicular monoamine transporter (VMAT). Furthermore, some Ca^{2+} is stored in specialized structures of the cell (Ca^{2+} stores). From these Ca^{2+} stores, Ca^{2+} can be released which increases the free Ca^{2+}. H₃-histamine receptor stimulation would reduce the release of Ca^{2+} from these stores and would thence reduce exocytosis of NE. Moreover, H₃-histamine receptors may stimulate sodium channels (NaC) in the cell and via the open NaC more Na^+ enters the cell. In addition, H₃-histamine receptor stimulation can inactivate phospholipase C (PLC) which would reduce PKC activity and this would reduce the activity of the sodium hydrogen antiporter (NHE): less sodium ions would enter the cell. H₃-histamine receptor stimulation can activate cGMP-dependent protein kinases (PKG) and the phosphoinositol-3-kinase (PI3 kinase). The latter would phosphorylate and activate protein kinase B (Akt) which in turn would phosphorylate and activate a phosphodiesterase 3 (PDE 3). PDE3 would then degrade cAMP faster leading to lower levels of cAMP and this would reduce the activity of PKA and therefore less exocytosis of NE would ensue. Conceivably, via β-arrestin H₃-histamine receptors can activate MAPK by increasing their phosphorylation state (modified from Panula et al. 2015, Levi and Smith 2005).

There are in vitro data with synaptic preparations from the human heart which show that histamine via stimulation of H₃-histamine receptors in hypoxic conditions (to simulate myocardial infarction) reduced the detrimental release of noradrenaline from synaptic preparations (Hatta et al. 1997). Global ischemia was repeatedly shown to cause increased density and degranulation of cardiac mast cells which would be an obvious source of histamine. Fittingly, in mast cell deficient mice, the extent of necrosis was lower than in WT mice, consistent with a detrimental role of mast cells (Levick et al. 2011).

In rejection of cardiac transplantations, histamine is known to increase in the plasma of patients (Moore et al. 1968, Dy et al. 1981). This process might involve the activation of cardiac mast cells and indeed in rejected hearts more activated mast cells were reported (Levick et al. 2011).

In a rat model of cardiac impairment (injection of isoproterenol), which led to cardiac infarction, a beneficial effect injection of a H_3-histamine receptor agonist (imetit) was noted (Hass et al. 2016).

12. Sepsis

In animal studies, sepsis was accompanied by hugely increased levels of histamine in the plasma (e.g., rabbits: Matsuda et al. 2002). There are animal studies that see detrimental effects of histamine in sepsis: in rats where sepsis was induced by injection of endotoxins. Here, additional injections of H_1-histamine receptor antagonists and H_2-histamine receptor antagonists increased the survival of the animals, suggesting that stimulation of H_1-histamine receptor and H_2-histamine receptor mediated some of the deadly effects of sepsis (Brackett et al. 1985). It is questionable how these findings can be translated to patients because as described above rats do not exhibit functional H_1-histamine receptor or H_2-histamine receptor in the cardiomyocyte but probably only in the vasculature. Moreover, and difficult to understand, inhibition of histamine metabolism by inhibiting histamine-N-methyl-transferase by amodaiquine reduced the mortality in mice: this was explained by protection of liver function (Yokoyama et al. 2007). H_2-histamine receptors on leucocytes inhibit neutrophil activation, superoxide that is free radical production, syntheses of luekotriene4 (Seligmann et al. 1983, Flamand et al. 2004, Carlos et al. 2013). H_4-histamine receptors on neutrophils inhibit degranulation (Dib et al. 2014). LPS increased the expression of H_1-histamine receptors and H_2-histamine receptors in the heart of rabbits with experimental sepsis (Matsuda et al. 2002). In another protocol of sepsis, a H_2-histamine receptor antagonist or in H_2-histamine receptor KO mice or HDC KO increased mortality of mice compared to wild type animals was reported (Yokoyama et al. 2004). This was interpreted that H_2-histamine receptors are detrimental in sepsis. They interpreted these data that LPS would induce the synthesis of histamine in Kupffer cells in the liver and this histamine would inhibit via H_2-histamine receptors the inflammation via reduction of the production of cytokines (Yokoyama et al. 2004). On the other hand, sepsis might in truth also involve H_3-histamine receptors. After LPS treatment, the contractility of the dogs was improved when they were pretreated with H_3-histamine receptor antagonists (Li et al. 1998). This was interpreted that histamine via H_3-histamine receptors acted by reducing cardiac preload (Li et al. 1998). They also argued that H_3-histamine receptors might be the first receptor to be activated when LPS increased histamine levels because the H_3-histamine receptor exhibits a higher affinity than H_1-histamine receptors and H_2-histamine receptors which is a valid point (Table 1, Li et al. 1998). Another mechanism might contribute to the detrimental effects of histamine in sepsis: in HUVECs LPS in vitro elevated COX2 expression and this increase was enhanced by histamine acting on H_1-histamine receptors (Tan et al. 2007). More recently it was shown that in a model of fecal sepsis, substantial amounts of bacteria that induced sepsis pass from the lymphatic system of the gut to the lung and liver (Assimakopoulos et al. 2018). Here, the integrity of cellular barriers in the gut and lymphatic system is crucial and these barriers might be broken by histamine receptors stimulation (Assimakopoulos et al. 2018). Furthermore, the cardiodepression in sepsis was suggested to be due to histamine-induced stimulation of H_3-histamine receptors in a canine model (Li et al. 1998). In isolated trabeculae from dog ventricle, the positive inotropic effect of field stimulation (prolonged duration of electrical stimulus) was blocked by propranolol indicating that released noradrenaline has acted on β-adrenoceptors. Moreover, 1 nM histamine also reduced the increase in force due to field stimulation and this effect was mimicked by a H_3-histamine receptor agonist and blocked by a H_3-histamine receptor antagonist (Li et al. 1998) and likewise, when septic serum extracts were added to canine trabeculae, a decrease in force was noted that was reversed by clobenpropit: thence, it was suggested that in human sepsis histamine via H_3-histamine receptors and pertussis toxin-sensitive GTP binding proteins might likewise block the positive inotropic function of noradrenaline released from ganglia in the heart (Li et al. 1998, Cheng et al. 2002). Histamine might play a detrimental role in sepsis because inflammation markers after experimental sepsis are lower and mortality is minor in HDC KO mice than in WT mice (Hattori et al. 2016). H_2-histamine receptor overexpression plays a detrimental role in LPS induced sepsis at least in mice

(Gergs et al. 2020a) and this finding supports previous work where H_2-histamine receptor KO mice (H_1-histamine receptor and H_2-histamine receptor double KO were studied) fared better in experimental sepsis (Hattori et al. 2016). Hence, animal (mouse) data suggest that a combined treatment with H_1-histamine receptor and H_2-histamine receptor antagonist might be helpful in clinical sepsis (Hattori et al. 2016).

13. Arrhythmias

In cavian ventricular cardiomyocytes histamine, (0.3 µM) stimulated the delayed potassium ion current via ranitidine-sensitive H_2-histamine receptors and this effect was attenuated by 1 µM carbachol (an unselective muscarinic receptor agonist) whereas less histamine (10-8 M) is sufficient to stimulate calcium ion currents (Borchard and Hafner 1986, Hescheler et al. 1987, Tanaka et al. 1991). This finding has been used to explain (Tanaka et al. 1991) why low concentrations of histamine can prolong the duration of cardiac action potentials (Eckel et al. 1982) whereas higher concentrations of histamine would shorten (Houki 1973, Senges et al. 1977, Ledda et al. 1977) the duration of monophasic cardiac action potentials. A shortening of the action potential might also follow from the reported histamine-induced increase in chloride anion currents in cardiac preparations. Some human data are available: early on intravenous injection or infusion of histamine led to multiple conduction irregularities like AV block of the third degree and irregular idioventricular rhythm (Schenk et al. 1921, Vigorito et al. 1983). In an US American study of patients presenting in the emergency ward with symptoms of acute allergic reactions, there was a positive correlations between arrhythmias in these patients and the plasma values of histamine (Lin et al. 2000). At the bulk of patients (60 from 66 patients) reacted allergic against food, the remainder medicinal drugs were suspected (Lin et al. 2000). A well-documented case of food poisoning (not food allergy but mechanistically relevant) led to AV block (Wansa et al. 2018). A 69 year old female had ingested spoiled mussels for dinner and was brought to a clinic where the ECG detected a complete atrioventricular block (Wansa et al. 2018). The patient complained of syncope (Wansa et al. 2018). The ECG alterations were explained by histamine formed in spoiled mussels reaching the heart and acting to block AV conduction by stimulation of H_1-histamine receptors (Wansa et al. 2018). In the pressure overloaded heart (induced by transverse aortic constriction) of mice, the incidence of inducible atrial arrhythmias increased and correlated with mast cell infiltration in these hearts. Hence, mediators of arrhythmias might be present in the heart: this could be histamine or platelet derived growth factor A (PDGF-A, Liao et al. 2010).

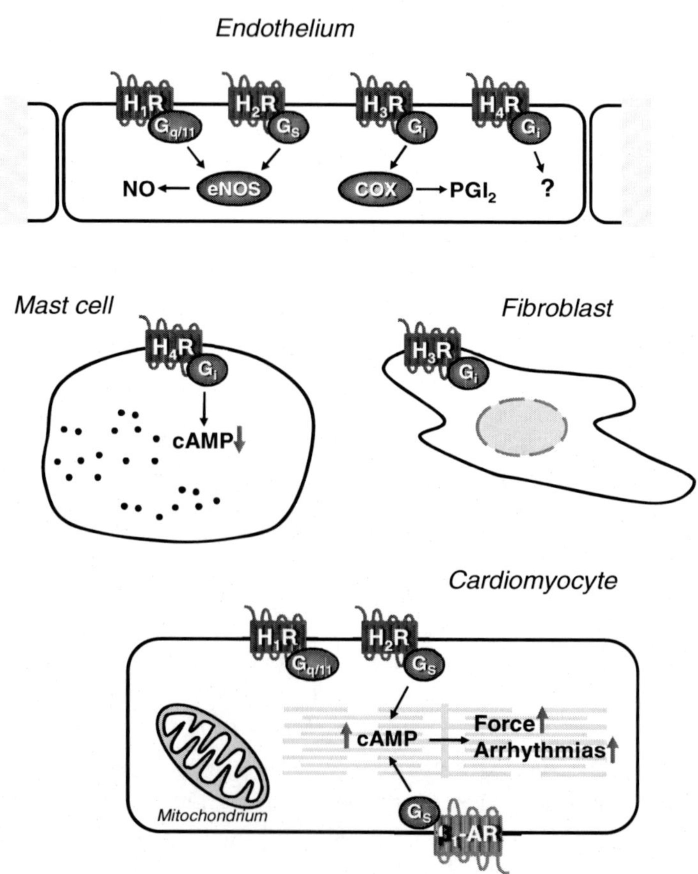

Figure 6. Here, the current view of cardiac expression of histamine receptors (H$_{1-4}$R) in the main cells of the heart is put together in more detail than in Figure 4. In the cardiac endothelium, all four histamine receptors are present, but only the function of H$_1$R and H$_2$R that lead via NO to vasodilation (see Figure 7) is really understood. H$_3$R lead to the production of vasodilatory prostaglandins (see Figure 7). Mast cells are present in cardiac tissue and express at least H$_4$R that reduce cAMP levels in the mast cell via inhibitory GTP-binding proteins (Gi) which reduces the release of histamine from the mast cell. On fibroblasts, H$_3$R are present and are thought to induce extrusion of proteins connected with fibrosis. Cardiomyocytes contain probably only H$_1$R and H$_2$R. H$_2$R probably use the same second messenger, cAMP, as the β-adrenoceptor. The H$_2$R like the β-adrenoceptors can increase force of contraction, but also can lead to detrimental cardiac arrhythmias.

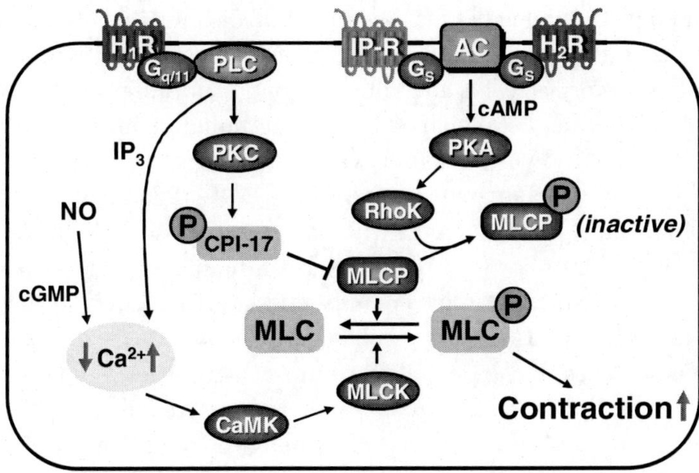

Figure 7. Here, a smooth muscle cell is shown in larger scale than in Figure 4. H₁R stimulation on smooth muscle cells leads via $G_{q/11}$ and phospholipase C (PLC) to activation of a protein kinase C (PKC) which produces inositol-tri-phosphate (IP₃) that finally induces an increase in free Ca^{2+}. This Ca^{2+} binds to calmodulin and activates a calcium/calmodulin dependent protein kinase (CaMK) that phosphorylates and activates a myosin light chain kinase (MLCK). The MLCK phosphorylates the myosin light chains (MLC) and this leads to smooth muscle contraction. This process is amplified because PLC also activates PKC which phosphorylates CPI-17 which then inhibits myosin light chain phosphatase (MLCP) and this also increases the phosphorylation state of MLC and thus contributes to contraction. On the other hand, there are H₂R on smooth muscle cells. Their stimulation increases cAMP levels in the smooth muscle cell. The generated cAMP augments the activity of the cAMP dependent protein kinase (PKA). PKA phosphorylates and activates another protein called RhoK. This can now lead to dephosphorylation of MLC and thence relaxation. In addition, PKA may reduce the free Ca^{2+} in the smooth muscle cells, also leading to relaxation. Moreover, nitric oxide, originating in endothelial cells (Figure 6) can enter the smooth muscle cell, and reduce free Ca^{2+} which will contribute to smooth muscle relaxation. Furthermore, the prostaglandin PGI₂ from endothelial cells (Figure 4, 6) increase cAMP content and induce relaxation via IP₃-R.

These reports are preliminary evidence that increase histamine due to allergies can lead to cardiac arrhythmias in man and is an important starting point for further research.

H₂-histamine receptor antagonists have been shown to reduce arrhythmias at least in isolated rabbit hearts (Frommeyer et al. 2017). In some case reports arrhythmias seem to be caused by histamine containing food (fish, Kiwi fruits: Rojas-Perez-Ezquerra et al. 2017). There is some evidence in mice that mast cells do not contribute at least to reperfusion arrhythmias (He et al. 2012). In contrast, mastocytosis, a disease with increased density of mast cell, has been reported to correlate and perhaps cause arrhythmias in adults and children

(Rohr et al. 2005, Shaffer et al. 2006); hence species difference might be relevant. In addition, mast cells in the heart are found in the vicinity of nerve fibers and thus histamine has a short way of diffusion (Reid et al. 2011).

On the other hand, histamine can induce vasoconstriction via H_1-histamine receptors and this can cause arrhythmias (reviewed by Wolff and Levi 1986). This can be explained because histamine which usually leads to vasodilation is known to cause vasoconstriction in epicardial human coronaries even in healthy persons (Ginsburg et al. 1981, 1984a, b). This can occur for instance if patients react with anaphylaxis against iodine containing contrast media for radiography (Simons and Simons 2011). Apparently large amounts of releasable histamine are present in arteries mainly located in mast cells. If in disease in patients or mechanically in animals the endothelial cells have been damaged, then released histamine can constrict coronary arteries in a potent way; this vasoconstriction was antagonized by an H_1-histamine receptor blocker and was thus classified as H_1-histamine receptor mediated (pig: Shimokawa et al. 1983; man: Ginsburg et al. 1981). It is possible that some types of Prinzmetal angina are cause by histamine (Kritikou et al. 2016). Overexpression of the H_2-histamine receptors alone and also their stimulation by agonists induce atrial and ventricular arrhythmia in mice which are abrogated by cimetidine, suggesting that increased expression of H_2-histamine receptors in human hearts might lead to atrial fibrillation or ventricular arrhythmias (Gergs et al. 2021). However, to the best of our knowledge expression of H_2-histamine receptors in cardiac tissue of patients with arrhythmias has not yet been published. Maybe register studies could be performed to find out whether antagonists at H_2-histamine receptors reduce the incidence of arrhythmias of any kind compared to a case control group.

14. Anaphylaxis

One has coined the term cardiac anaphylaxis to sum up the effects of release of histamine following an antigenic reaction by mast cells in basophils in patients (Bani et al. 2006). Anaphylactic reactions can occur in the cardiovascular system and their symptoms included tachycardia, hypotension and finally cardiac shock (Kaliner et al. 1981). In vitro, in animal experiments, one can release histamine in mast cells from the heart of animals sensitized for instance against ovalbumin (Penna et al. 1959, Felix et al. 1988). The usual explanation is a follows: mast cells contain histamine granules and mast cells release histamine via IgE-dependent degranulation. The crosslinking of IgE antibodies bound to the IgE receptors after FceRI exposure to allergens, lead to activation of a tyrosine kinase, of phospholipase C, of protein kinase C and then to a Ca^{2+} increase that induces via phosphorylation of proteins the degranulation of the mast cells (Hirasawa 2019). This leads to increased production of immunoglobulin E in mast cells and sensitization of mast cells and basophils (Hirasawa 2019). Exposure to the allergen released histamine (and other mediators) from these sensitized cells. Then, action of histamine on its receptors induced the cardiovascular events mentioned above. These reactions in guinea pig hearts were antagonized by a H_1-histamine receptor blocker but not by a H_2-histamine receptor blocker in some studies (Felix et al. 1991). Others reported that H_2-histamine receptor blockers impaired the release of histamine from mast cells (Blandina et al. 1987). Histamine and H_2-histamine receptor agonists can abrogate the release of histamine from mast cells via stimulation of H_2-histamine receptors (Blandina et al. 1987). Allergen-induced release of histamine from the heart is stimulated by noradrenaline via α_1-adrenoceptors (Giotti et al. 1966). As H_3-histamine receptor stimulation has been reported to reduce release of noradrenaline from cardiac ganglia, this reduction of noradrenaline might lead to less allergic histamine release and thus H_3-histamine receptors might be beneficial in cardiac allergy (Endou et al. 1994). The putative role of histamine in cardiac anaphylaxis is in line with the observation that addition of a histamine degrading enzyme from plants to sensitized hearts reduces not only histamine levels in cardiac effluates but also the above mentioned allergic induced increase in force and heartbeat in the cavian heart (Masini et al. 2002). If histamine is released in an anaphylactic reaction against a venom, cardiac arrhythmias have been described (see below under Arrhythmias for details, Kounis et al. 2019). In an emergency ward study, mainly allergic reactions against shellfish, fish, fruit and tree nuts were reported (Lin et al. 2000). From their anamnesis, a minority of patients was allergic against medicinal drugs and one out of 66 against a recreational drug (Lin et al. 2000). As concerns medicinal drugs, studies have identified vancomycin (red man syndrome), anesthetic drugs (Cottinau et al. 1996) and radiocontrast material (Renz et al. 1998) as potential allergens. Death following allergic reactions to food, anesthetic drugs and radiocontrast material is still observed today (Esposito et al. 2021). Hymenoptera sting is also known to lead to allergies correlated with elevated plasma histamine levels (van der Linden et al. 1992). The use of histamine antagonists or mast cell stabilizers to treat arrhythmias in allergic and atopic patients has been suggested (Layfritz et al. 2014).

15. Heart Failure

An important cause of heart failure beyond any doubt is long standing hypertension. Plasma of patients with chronic hypertension contained less histamine in the plasma than normotensive patients. Hence, histamine has been suggested to act as an endogenous blood pressure lowering agent because of its dilatory effects on arterial vessels (Campos et al. 1999). In addition, histamine via H_1-histamine receptors at least in HUVEC increased the expression eNOS which would via NO formation further reduced blood pressure (Li et al. 2003). In patients with heart failure, the activity of DAO is increased (Stolen et al. 2004). There is evidence that the positive inotropic effect of histamine via H_2-histamine receptors is not impaired in heart failure patients (Bristow et al. 1982a, Baumann et al. 1984). This looks beneficial at first glance; the same group has recently interpreted their data in a different way: this sustained coupling of the H_2-histamine receptor to cAMP generation might detrimentally lead to arrhythmias as all cAMP elevating agents via an increase in cellular Ca^{2+} can lead to depolarization and arrhythmias (Leary et al. 2018). This interpretation followed a clinical study where the H_2-histamine receptor antagonist famotidine could reduce the incidence of cardiac hypertrophy in patients over several years (Leary et al. 2018). In fairness, one has to consider that another group reported the opposite: a reduced positive inotropic effect of histamine in heart failure patients; of course, the different clinical data or different methodology might explain this discrepancy (Brown et al. 1986, Böhm et al. 1988). In patients with overt heart failure or idiopathic cardiomyopathy, elevated plasma histamine levels have been reported (Zdravkovic et al. 2011, Chen et al. 2017). The density of mast cells in the heart increased in patient with heart failure (Patella et al. 1998). This histamine may be released and might act on histamine receptors to increase cardiac fibrosis in heart failure patients (Patella et al. 1998). In a study on Han Chinese patients, one noted a positive correlation of heart failure and the expression of H_3-histamine receptors but not H_2-histamine receptors (or DAO or HMT: He et al. 2016), suggesting a role of the H_3-histamine receptor in the many steps in the pathogenesis of heart failure.

It is an unsolved clinical problem that the antitumor drug doxorubicin leads to heart failure in a many patients. This doxorubicin-induced heart failure was accompanied in studies with dogs to elevated histamine levels which have been claimed to contribute the doxorubicin-induced heart failure (Bristow et al. 1981). Later, similar data were obtained in rats: doxorubicin increased histamine concentrations in the rat heart (Decorti et al. 1997). More recent data argue quite oppositely; histamine is not a cause of heart failure in doxorubicin treated patients but may be a self-defense mechanism. This hypothesis is based on the following findings: injection of histamine together with doxorubicin reduced in comparison to injection of doxorubicin alone the severity of cardiac damage which was explained by beneficial effects of H_3-histamine receptor and H_4-histamine receptor stimulation by reducing of noradrenaline, arrhythmias and fibrosis (Martinel Lamas et al. 2015).

Experimental induced heart failure in dogs (mitral valve insufficiency) led to an increase of the density of mast cells in the hearts and could be attenuated by cromoglicic acid, a compound that inhibits the release of histamine from mast cells (Levick et al. 2008). In H_2-histamine receptor KO mice, aortic banding led to less cardiac hypertrophy and was thus interpreted as evidence for the detrimental role of histamine acting via H_2-histamine receptors (Zeng et al. 2014). Cardiac overexpression of H_2-histamine receptors in the mouse heart protected the ventricular function in a genetic model of cardiac hypertrophy and failure (Gergs et al. 2020b).

Very recent data point into another direction: one used an animal model of cardiorenal syndrome where angiotensin II was given, a nephrectomy was performed and high salt was given (=ANS). Animals exhibited high blood pressure and consecutively heart failure with cardiac hypertrophy and cardiac fibrosis and elevation (about 2.6 fold) of plasma histamine levels (Noguchi et al. 2020). The phenotype deteriorated if animals with ablation of HDC were used, suggesting to the authors a protective role of histamine (Noguchi et al. 2020). Alternatively, if ANS mice were treated with H_3-histamine receptor blockers, their renal and cardiac function deteriorated but not when H_1-histamine receptor blockers or H_2-histamine receptor blockers were given, suggesting a protective role of H_3-histamine receptors in this model (Noguchi et al. 2020). Indeed, beneficial effects of H_3-histamine receptor agonism was noted (Noguchi et al. 2020). They used immetridine as an H_3-histamine receptor agonist and this compound reduced the mRNA of genes related to inflammation (Noguchi et al. 2020).

16. Drug Interactions

In the isolated perfused cavian hearts, a detrimental interaction of ouabain (a cardiac glycoside) and histamine was reported: ouabain increased histamine induced AV block (Levi and Pappano 1972). Hence, it is conceivable, but was apparently never studied, that in patients with elevated histamine levels (possibly due to elevated levels of mast cells) digoxin has more unwanted proarrhythmic effects. Prolonged treatment of patients with β-adrenoceptor agonists led in vitro to a higher incidence of arrhythmias presumably via H_2-histamine receptor stimulation (Sanders et al. 1996). Whether this occurs clinically has apparently never been reported.

Interference with histamine degradation can lead to higher levels of histamine in the blood and thus to histamine induced side effects like tachycardia or flush. Such an interaction was reported for the antibiotic drug pentamidine which inhibits DAO activity in man (Mc Grath et al. 2010). In the same way, by inhibition of DAO activity, also cimetidine, dihydralazine and diphenhydramine could increase plasma levels of histamine (Wantke et al. 1998). Even red wine contains DAO inhibitors (besides alcohol) and thence, red wine induced arrhythmias might in part actually be due to enhanced histamine levels in the plasma (Maintz et al. 2006, Schirone et al. 2016). In addition, not only red wine but also other food like some sorts of fish, old cheese or some fruits (kiwi) contain high amounts of histamine (in part because of microbial activity) as well as ingredients that lead to inhibition of the activity of DAO. This is then thought to explain the allergic response to these kinds of food but also cardiac tachycardia or other arrhythmias (Maintz et al. 2006, Schirone et al. 2016). It is also known that degradation of histamine by histamine methyl transferase is blocked by diphenhydramine and other H_1-histamine receptor antagonists. In this way, diphenhydramine might attenuate its own action as a H_1-histamine receptor antagonist: it increases the plasma levels of histamine (Adachi et al. 2011). There is at least a positive correlation between increased plasma levels of histamine and increased incidences of arrhythmias (Layritz et al. 2014). Phosphodiesterase inhibitors potentiated the positive inotropic effects of histamine in a mouse model of cardiac H_2-histamine receptor overexpression (Neumann et al. 2021b). There are case reports that injection but also oral administration of antagonists at H_2-histamine-receptors (cimetidine, ranitidine and famotidine) lead to partial or complete atrioventricular blocks but also to fatal cardiac arrest which are explained by endogenous histamine acting on H_1-histamine receptors in the atrioventricular node cells to inhibit conduction or impaired coronary dilatation due to blockage of vasodilatory H_2-histamine-receptors, prolactin release or cholinergic effects (e.g., famotidine: Schoenwald et al. 1999). The package labeling warns physicians that bradycardia and/or AV blocks can occur with injection of antagonists at H_2-histamine-receptors (Schoenwald et al. 1999). Surprisingly, two antiarrhythmic drugs that are amiodarone and lorcainide are antagonists at H_3-histamine receptors which is not thought to contribute to their antiarrhythmic action but may be an untoward effect (Del Tredici et al. 2013).

17. Psychiatric Drugs

It is well known that many antidepressant and antipsychotic drugs block H_1-histamine receptors in the CNS and this is thought to underlie the body weight enhancing and sedative effect of these drugs. H_1-histamine receptor blockers are available in many countries without a prescription and they are very often used by patients (Simons and Simons 2011). One can hypothesize that these H_1-histamine receptor antagonist act on the heart and might increase the beating rate because the conduction slowing effects of H_1-histamine receptors in the human AV node are reduced. Some data to that effect have been reported (Abernathy et al. 2017). However, one has to keep in mind that H_1-histamine receptor blockers like terfenadine also block potassium channel and that has been thought to lead to deathly torsade be pointes arrhythmias (Panula et al. 2015). More to the point, cetirizine does not block potassium channels but can induce arrhythmias, which is easily explained by overweight of histamine induced H_2-histamine receptor stimulation (Abajo and Rodruigez 1999). The role of H_2-histamine receptors in the human AV node is not fully understood. However, H_2-histamine receptor blockers like ranitidine and famotidine have been reported clinically to lead to AV blocks and this could be explained by block of AV node cells (Allegri et al. 1988, Schoenwald et al. 1999). On the other hand, terfenadine and astemizole can release histamine from mast cells and this released histamine might induce unintended cardiovascular effects (Llenas et al. 1999).

Moreover, many antidepressant and antipsychotic drugs do not only block H_1-histamine receptors, as mentioned above, but also block at therapeutic drug concentrations H_2-histamine receptors (Amitriptyline, Imipramine: Appl et al. 2012 for data at recombinant human H_1-histamine receptors, H_2-histamine receptors, H_3-histamine receptors and H_4-histamine receptors). For instance, clozapine blocked human cardiac H_2 receptors in bindings studies (Appl et al. 2012, Hubert-Claude et al. 2012) and can also block the function of the human H_2-histamine receptor on contractility (unpublished observations from our group). Lysergic acid diethylamide (LSD) acted as a partial agonist in the heart: LSD has been noted to antagonize the positive inotropic effect of histamine in isolated cavian ventricular preparations and a biphasic initial positive chronotropic than negative chronotropic on cavian right atrial preparations (Angus and Black 1980). Initial data detected that LSD exerts agonistic positive inotropic effects in left atrial and ventricular preparations of H_2-histamine receptor overexpressing mice and that LSD at least in the presence of the phosphodiesterase inhibitors cilostamide and rolipram augments force of contraction in isolated right atrial preparations from patients (unpublished observations from our group).

The newer atypical antipsychotic drug olanzapine also blocks H_3- and H_4-histamine receptors (Appl et al. 2012). One can hypothesize that a several month long block of H_2-histamine receptors by amitriptyline might lead to upregulation of H_2-histamine receptors. A long period of treatment is typical for antidepressant drugs because it usually takes more than four weeks to notice an improvement of the depression in patients. If then amitriptyline intake is rapidly stopped, H_2-histamine receptor mediated side effects could be predicted. Indeed, amitriptyline could attenuate the inotropic and chronotropic effects of histamine in a mouse with cardiac overexpression of H_2-histamine receptors and also in human atrial muscle strips (Neumann et al. 2021b). Also, the long term treatment with olanzapine would be predicted to lead to a compensatory increase in H_4-histamine receptor density. If then olanzapine is not more given, an unintended overstimulation of cardiac H_4-histamine receptors is conceivable with more inhibition of noradrenaline release even under physiological conditions.

18. Genetic Models

Here, we have put together genetic mouse models that have been used or could be used in the research to understand histamine function better in the heart. It is questionable that H_1-histamine receptor or H_2-histamine receptor floxed mice would be of easily understandable usefulness, as histamine itself seems not to act via H_1-histamine receptors or H_2-histamine receptors in wild type mice (Gergs et al. 2019, 2020). However, a role for H_3-histamine receptors and H_4-histamine receptors at least in ischemia and reperfusion was demonstrated in wild type hearts and these effects were lacking in H_3-histamine receptor or H_4-histamine receptor KO hearts. Hence, it would be interesting to test in mice with a nerve cell or mast cell specific knock out, which can be easily generated if floxed H_3-histamine receptor and H_4-histamine receptor mice are available by crossbreeding with mice that express a CRE-activity only in nerve cells or mast cells. A cardiac phenotype of histamine N-methyl-transferase has apparently not been studied. The cardiac function of HDC KO mice was reported but it is difficult to compare with humans because mice have no functional cardiac H_2-histamine receptors. To address this topic properly, one would simply have to crossbreed HDC KO and H_2-histamine receptor overexpressing mice: in these mice one could elegantly study the role of HDC for cardiac histamine production. As a confirmatory study, one could use HDC-Cre mice crossbred with a fluorescence-protein-reporter mouse: this has been successfully used to study the presence of HDC in cells of the gastrointestinal tract and the brain (Walker et al. 2013). Apparently, in this elegant study, one did not look for HDC expression in the heart that is in which cells of the heart, HDC is actually expressed (Walker et al. 2013). Such data are expected with interest. Moreover, recently a floxed HDC mouse have been generated: therefore, it should now be possible to ablate HDC only in cardiomyocytes (or other cardiac cells) at will, and thus it would be possible to study how relevant HDC in cardiomyocytes and therefore histamine production in cardiomyocytes really is for cardiac function. For completeness and in order to facilitate to the reader to plan experiments, in last column of Table 6, typical organic molecules used in the field to inhibit these enzymes were also plotted.

Conclusion

Though cardiac action of histamine has now been studied for over 100 years, we still get more and deeper insight. Histamine plays a currently not exactly defined role in many cardiac diseases. We need to understand the pathophysiological role of histamine in the heart better to come up with new therapeutic concepts involving dungs that interfere with the formation, degradation and storage of histamine as well as agonists and antagonists on the four canonical histamine receptors. Using new genetic models in combination seems to open some fruitful paths to progress in cardiology.

References

Abajo FJ and Rodriguez LA. Risk of ventricular arrhythmias associated with nonsedating antihistamine drugs. *Br J Clin Pharmacol* 1999 47:307-313.
Abernathy A, Alsina L, Greer J, Egerman R. Transient Fetal Tachycardia After Intravenous Diphenhydramine Administration. *Obstet Gynecol.* 2017 Aug;130(2):374-376.

Adachi N, Itoh Y, Oishi R, Saeki K. Direct evidence for increased continuous histamine release in the striatum of conscious freely moving rats produced by middle cerebral artery occlusion. *J Cereb Blood Flow Metab.* 1992 May;12(3):477-83.

Adachi N, Liu K, Ninomiya K, Matsuoka E, Motoki A, Irisawa Y, Nishibori M. Reduction of the infarct size by simultaneous administration of L-histidine and diphenhydramine in ischaemic rat brains. *Resuscitation.* 2011 Feb;82(2):219-21.

Adderley SP, Lawrence C, Madonia E, Olubadewo JO, Breslin JW. Histamine activates p38 MAP kinase and alters local lamellipodia dynamics, reducing endothelial barrier integrity and eliciting central movement of actin fibers. *Am J Physiol Cell Physiol.* 2015 Jul 1;309(1):C51-9. doi: 10.1152/ajpcell.00096.2015.

Aldi S, Takano K, Tomita K, Koda K, Chan NY, Marino A, Salazar-Rodriguez M, Thurmond RL, Levi R. Histamine H4-receptors inhibit mast cell renin release in ischemia/reperfusion via protein kinase C ε-dependent aldehyde dehydrogenase type-2 activation. *J Pharmacol Exp Ther.* 2014 Jun;349(3):508-17.

Allegri G, Pellegrini K, Dobrilla G. First-degree atrioventricular block in a young duodenal ulcer patient treated with a standard oral dose of ranitidine. *Agents Actions.* 1988 Jul;24(3-4):237-42.

Angus JA, Black JW. Pharmacological assay of cardiac H2-receptor blockade by amitriptyline and lysergic acid diethylamide. *Circ Res.* 1980 Jun;46(6 Pt 2):I64-9.

Appl H, Holzammer T, Dove S, Haen E, Strasser A, Seifert R. Interactions of recombinant human histamine H1R, H2R, H3R, and H4R receptors with 34 antidepressants and antipsychotics. *Naunyn-Schmiedebergs Arch Pharmacol.* 2012 Feb;385(2):145-70.

Asanuma H, Minamino T, Ogai A, Kim J, Asakura M, Komamura K, Sanada S, Fujita M, Hirata A, Wakeno M, Tsukamoto O, Shinozaki Y, Myoishi M, Takashima S, Tomoike H, Kitakaze M. Blockade of histamine H2 receptors protects the heart against ischemia and reperfusion injury in dogs. *J Mol Cell Cardiol.* 2006 May;40(5):666-74.

Assimakopoulos SF, Triantos C, Thomopoulos K, Fligou F, Maroulis I, Marangos M, Gogos CA. Gut-origin sepsis in the critically ill patient: pathophysiology and treatment. *Infection.* 2018 Dec;46(6):751-760. doi: 10.1007/s15010-018-1178-5.

Bani D, Nistri S, Mannaioni PF, Masini E. Cardiac anaphylaxis: pathophysiology and therapeutic perspectives. *Curr Allergy Asthma Rep.* 2006 Feb;6(1):14-9. doi: 10.1007/s11882-006-0004-9.

Barger G, Ewins AJ. Some phenolic derivatives of β-phenylethylamine. *Journal of the Chemical Society Transactions,* 1910, 2253- 2261.

Bartlet AL. The action of histamine in the isolated heart. *Br J Pharmacol Chemother.* 1963 Dec;21:450-61.

Baumann G, Permanetter B, Wirtzfeld A. Possible value of H2-receptor agonists for treatment of catecholamine-insensitive congestive heart failure. *Pharmacol Ther.* 1984;24(2):165-77.

Benedetti MS, Ancher JF, Sontag N. Monoamine oxidase inhibitors and histamine metabolism. *Experientia.* 1980 Jul 15;36(7):818-10. doi: 10.1007/BF0 1978589.

Best CH, Dale HH, Dudley HW, Thorpe WV. The nature of the vaso-dilator constituents of certain tissue extracts. *J Physiol.* 1927 Mar 15;62(4):397-417.

Bhardwaj RK, Herrera-Ruiz D, Eltoukhy N, Saad M, Knipp GT. The functional evaluation of human peptide/histidine transporter 1 (hPHT1) in transiently transfected COS-7 cells. *Eur J Pharm Sci.* 2006 Apr;27(5):533-42. doi: 10.1016/j.ejps.2005.09.014.

Black JW, Duncan WA, Durant CJ, Ganellin CR, Parsons EM. Definition and antagonism of histamine H 2 -receptors. *Nature.* 1972 Apr 21;236(5347):385-90. doi: 10.1038/236385a0.

Blandina P, Brunelleschi S, Fantozzi R, Giannella E, Mannaioni PF, Masini E. The antianaphylactic action of histamine H2-receptor agonists in the guinea-pig isolated heart. *Br J Pharmacol.* 1987 Mar;90(3):459-66. doi: 10.1111/j.1476-5381.1987.tb11195.x.

Böhm M, Beuckelmann D, Brown L, Feiler G, Lorenz B, Näbauer M, Kemkes B, Erdmann E. Reduction of beta-adrenoceptor density and evaluation of positive inotropic responses in isolated, diseased human myocardium. *Eur Heart J.* 1988 Aug;9(8):844-52.

Bono P, Jalkanen S, Salmi M. Mouse vascular adhesion protein 1 is a sialoglycoprotein with enzymatic activity and is induced in diabetic insulitis. *Am J Pathol.* 1999 Nov;155(5):1613-24.

Boomsma F, van Veldhuisen DJ, de Kam PJ, Man in't Veld AJ, Mosterd A, Lie KI, Schalekamp MA. Plasma semicarbazide-sensitive amine oxidase is elevated in patients with congestive heart failure. *Cardiovasc Res.* 1997 Feb;33(2):387-91.

Borchard U, Hafner D. Electrophysiological characterization of histamine receptor subtypes in mammalian heart preparations. *Naunyn Schmiedebergs Arch Pharmacol.* 1986 Nov;334(3):294-302.

Brackett DJ, Schaefer CF, Wilson MF. The effects of H1 and H2 histamine receptor antagonists on the development of endotoxemia in the conscious, unrestrained rat. *Circ Shock.* 1985;16(2):141-53.

Bristow MR, Ginsburg R, Minobe W, Cubicciotti RS, Sageman WS, Lurie K, Billingham ME, Harrison DC, Stinson EB. Decreased catecholamine sensitivity and beta-adrenergic-receptor density in failing human hearts. *N Engl J Med.* 1982a Jul 22;307(4):205-11.

Bristow MR, Minobe WA, Billingham ME, Marmor JB, Johnson GA, Ishimoto BM, Sageman WS, Daniels JR. Anthracycline-associated cardiac and renal damage in rabbits. Evidence for mediation by vasoactive substances. *Lab Invest.* 1981 Aug;45(2):157-68.

Brown L, Lorenz B, Erdmann E. Reduced positive inotropic effects in diseased human ventricular myocardium. *Cardiovasc Res.* 1986 Jul;20(7):516-20.

Campos HA, Montenegro M, Velasco M, Romero E, Alvarez R, Urbina A. Treadmill exercise-induced stress causes a rise of blood histamine in normotensive but not in primary hypertensive humans. *Eur J Pharmacol.* 1999 Oct 21;383(1):69-73.

Carlos D, Spiller F, Souto FO, Trevelin SC, Borges VF, de Freitas A, Alves-Filho JC, Silva JS, Ryffel B, Cunha FQ. Histamine h2 receptor signaling in the pathogenesis of sepsis: studies in a murine diabetes model. *J Immunol.* 2013 Aug 1;191(3):1373-82. doi: 10.4049/jimmunol.1202907.

Cases O, Seif I, Grimsby J, Gaspar P, ChenK, et al. 1995. Aggressive behavior and al-tered amounts of brain serotonin and nore-pinephrine in mice lacking MAO A. *Science* 268(5218):1763–66.

Chan NY, Robador PA, Levi R. Natriuretic peptide-induced catecholamine release from cardiac sympathetic neurons: inhibition by histamine H3 and H4 receptor activation. *J Pharmacol Exp Ther.* 2012 Dec;343(3):568-77.

Chen J, Hong T, Ding S, Deng L, Abudupataer M, Zhang W, Tong M, Jia J, Gong H, Zou Y, Wang TC, Ge J, Yang X.Aggravated myocardial infarction-induced cardiac remodeling and heart failure in histamine-deficient mice. *Sci Rep.* 2017 Mar 8;7:44007.

Cheng ZQ, Bose D, Jacobs H, Light RB, Mink SN. Sepsis causes presynaptic histamine H3 and alpha2-adrenergic dysfunction in canine myocardium. *Cardiovasc Res.* 2002 Nov;56(2):225-34. doi: 10.1016/s0008-6363(02)00543-6.

Chiba S. Blocking effect of tripelennamine on histamine--induced positive chronotropic and inotropic responses of the dog atrium. *Tohoku J Exp Med.* 1976 Nov;120(3):299-300.

Coelho MH, Silva IJ, Azevedo MS, Manso CF. Decrease in blood histamine in drug-treated parkinsonian patients. *Mol Chem Neuropathol.* 1991 Apr;14(2):77-85. doi: 10.1007/BF03159928.

Cottineau C, Drouet M, Costerousse F, Dussaussoy C, Sabbah A. Intérêt des médiateurs plasmatiques (histamine et tryptase) et urinaire (méthylhistamine) lors des réactions anaphylactiques et/ou anaphylactoïdes peranesthésiques

[Importance of plasma (histamine and tryptase) and urinary (methylhistamine) in peri-anesthetic anaphylactic and/or anaphylactoid reactions]. *Allerg Immunol* (Paris). 1996 Oct;28(8):270, 273-6.

Dai S. A study of the actions of histamine on the isolated rat heart. *Clin Exp Pharmacol Physiol.* 1976 Jul-Aug;3(4):359-67.

Dale HH, Laidlaw PP. The physiological action of beta-iminazolylethylamine. *J Physiol.* 1910 Dec 31;41(5):318-44.

Decorti G, Candussio L, Klugmann FB, Strohmayer A, Mucci MP, Mosco A, Baldini L. Adriamycin-induced histamine release from heart tissue in vitro. *Cancer Chemother Pharmacol.* 1997;40(4):363-6.

Del Tredici AL, Ma JN, Piu F, Burstein ES. Identification of the antiarrhythmic drugs amiodarone and lorcainide as potent H3 histamine receptor inverse agonists. *J Pharmacol Exp Ther.* 2014 Jan;348(1):116-24. doi: 10.1124/jpet.113.208892.

Del Valle J, Gantz I. Novel insights into histamine H2 receptor biology. *Am J Physiol.* 1997 Nov;273(5 Pt 1):G987-96.

Dib K, Perecko T, Jenei V, McFarlane C, Comer D, Brown V, Katebe M, Scheithauer T, Thurmond RL, Chazot PL, Ennis M. The histamine H4 receptor is a potent inhibitor of adhesion-dependent degranulation in human neutrophils. *J Leukoc Biol.* 2014 Sep;96(3):411-8. doi: 10.1189/jlb.2AB0813-432RR.

Du XY, Schoemaker RG, X462P6, Bos E, Saxena PR. Effects of histamine on porcine isolated myocardium: differentiation from effects on human tissue. *J Cardiovasc Pharmacol.* 1993 Sep;22(3):468-73. doi: 10.1097/00005344-199309000-00019.

Duan H, Wang J. Impaired monoamine and organic cation uptake in choroid plexus in mice with targeted disruption of the plasma membrane monoamine transporter (Slc29a4) gene. *J Biol Chem.* 2013 Feb 1;288(5):3535-44. doi: 10.1074/jbc.M112.436972.

Duan H, Wang J. Selective transport of monoamine neurotransmitters by human plasma membrane monoamine transporter and organic cation transporter 3. *J Pharmacol Exp Ther.* 2010 Dec;335(3):743-53.

Duicu OM, Lighezan R, Sturza A, Ceausu RA, Borza C, Vaduva A, Noveanu L, Gaspar M, Ionac A, Feier H, Muntean DM, Mornos C. Monoamine Oxidases as Potential Contributors to Oxidative Stress in Diabetes: Time for a Study in Patients Undergoing Heart Surgery. *Biomed Res Int.* 2015;2015:515437. doi: 10.1155/2015/515437.

Dy M, Lebel B, Kamoun P, Hamburger J. Histamine production during the anti-allograft response. Demonstration of a new lymphokine enhancing histamine synthesis. *J Exp Med.* 1981 Feb 1;153(2):293-309.

Dyer J, Warren K, Merlin S, Metcalfe DD, Kaliner M. Measurement of plasma histamine: description of an improved method and normal values. *J Allergy Clin Immunol.* 1982 Aug;70(2):82-7. doi: 10.1016/0091-6749(82)90233-0.

Ea Kim L, Javellaud J, Oudart N. Endothelium-dependent relaxation of rabbit middle cerebral artery to a histamine H3-agonist is reduced by inhibitors of nitric oxide and prostacyclin synthesis. *Br J Pharmacol.* 1992 Jan;105(1):103-6. doi: 10.1111/j.1476-5381.1992.tb14218.x.

Eckel L, Gristwood RW, Nawrath H, Owen DA, Satter P. Inotropic and electrophysiological effects of histamine on human ventricular heart muscle. *J Physiol.* 1982 Sep;330:111-23.

Ehrlich P. Beiträge zur Kenntnis dergranulirten Bindegewebszellen und der eosino-philen Leukocyten. *Arch. Anat. Physiol., Lpz.,* 1879; 3,166-169.

Elion GB, Kovensky A, Hitchings GH. Metabolic studies of allopurinol, an inhibitor of xanthine oxidase. *Biochem Pharmacol.* 1966 Jul;15(7):863-80. doi: 10.1016/0006-2952(66)90163-8.

Endo Y, Kumagai K. Induction by interleukin-1, tumor necrosis factor and lipopolysaccharides of histidine decarboxylase in the stomach and prolonged accumulation of gastric acid. *Br J Pharmacol.* 1998 Oct;125(4):842-8. doi: 10.1038/sj.bjp.0702108.

Endoh M. Correlation of cyclic AMP and cyclic GMP levels with changes in contractile force of dog ventricular myocardium during cholinergic antagonism of positive inotropic actions of histamine, glucagon, theophylline and papaverine. *Jpn J Pharmacol.* 1979 Dec;29(6):855-64.

Ercan-Sencicek AG, Stillman AA, Ghosh AK, Bilguvar K, O'Roak BJ, Mason CE, Abbott T, Gupta A, King RA, Pauls DL, Tischfield JA, Heiman GA, Singer HS, Gilbert DL, Hoekstra PJ, Morgan TM, Loring E, Yasuno K, Fernandez T, Sanders S, Louvi A, Cho JH, Mane S, Colangelo CM, Biederer T, Lifton RP, Gunel M, State MW.: L-histidine decarboxylase and Tourette syndrome. *N. Engl. J. Med.,* 2010; 362: 1901–1908.

Esposito M, Montana A, Liberto A, Filetti V, Nunno ND, Amico F, Salerno M, Loreto C, Sessa F. Anaphylactic Death: A New Forensic Workflow for Diagnosis. *Healthcare* (Basel). 2021 Jan 22;9(2):117. doi: 10.3390/healthcare9020117.

Eto M, Kitazawa T, Yazawa M, Mukai H, Ono Y, Brautigan DL. Histamine-induced vasoconstriction involves phosphorylation of a specific inhibitor protein for myosin phosphatase by protein kinase C alpha and delta isoforms. *J Biol Chem.* 2001 Aug 3;276(31):29072-8. doi: 10.1074/jbc.M103206200.

Felix SB, Baumann G, Helmus S, Sattelberger U. The role of histamine in cardiac anaphylaxis; characterization of histaminergic H1- and H2-receptor effects. *Basic Res Cardiol.* 1988 Sep-Oct;83(5):531-9. doi: 10.1007/BF01906682.

Felix SB, Buschauer A, Baumann G. Therapeutic value of H2-receptor stimulation in congestive heart failure. Hemodynamic effects of BU-E-76, BU-E-75 and arpromidine (BU-E-50) in comparison to impromidine. *Agents Actions Suppl.* 1991;33:257-69.

Ferstl R, Frei R, Barcik W, Schiavi E, Wanke K, Ziegler M, Rodriguez-Perez N, Groeger D, Konieczna P, Zeiter S, Nehrbass D, Lauener R, Akdis CA, O'Mahony L. Histamine receptor 2 modifies iNKT cell activity within the inflamed lung. *Allergy.* 2017 Dec;72(12):1925-1935. doi: 10.1111/all.13227.

Flamand N, Plante H, Picard S, Laviolette M, Borgeat P. Histamine-induced inhibition of leukotriene biosynthesis in human neutrophils: involvement of the H2 receptor and cAMP. *Br J Pharmacol.* 2004 Feb;141(4):552-61. doi: 10.1038/sj.bjp.0705654.

Frommeyer G, Sterneberg M, Dechering DG, Kaese S, Bögeholz N, Pott C, Fehr M, Bogossian Milberg P, Eckardt L. Effective suppression of atrial fibrillation by the antihistaminic agent antazoline: First experimental insights into a novel antiarrhythmic agent. *Cardiovasc Ther.* 2017 Apr;35(2).

Fühner H. Das Pituitrin und seine wirksamen Bestandteile. *Münchner Medizinische Wochenschrift* 1912 no 16: 852-3.

Fukushima Y, Shindo T, Anai M, Saitoh T, Wang Y, Fujishiro M, Ohashi Y, Ogihara T, Inukai K, Ono H, Sakoda H, Kurihara Y, Honda M, Shojima N, Fukushima H, Haraikawa-Onishi Y, Katagiri H, Shimizu Y, Ichinose M, Ishikawa T, Omata M, Nagai R, Kurihara H, Asano T. Structural and functional characterization of gastric mucosa and central nervous system in histamine H2 receptor-null mice. *Eur J Pharmacol.* 2003 May 2;468(1):47-58. doi: 10.1016/s0014-2999(03)01668-6.

Genovese A, Gross SS, Sakuma I, Levi R. Adenosine promotes histamine H1-mediated negative chronotropic and inotropic effects on human atrial myocardium. *J Pharmacol Exp Ther.* 1988 Dec;247(3):844-9.

Gergs U, Bernhardt G, Buchwalow IB, Edler H, Fröba J, Keller M, Kirchhefer U, Köhler F, Mißlinger N, Wache H, Neumann J. Initial Characterization of Transgenic Mice Overexpressing Human Histamine H2 Receptors. *J Pharmacol Exp Ther.* 2019 Apr;369(1):129-141. doi: 10.1124/jpet.118.255711.

Gergs U, Kirchhefer U, Bergmann F, Künstler B, Mißlinger N, Au B, Mahnkopf M, Wache H, Neumann J. Characterization of Stressed Transgenic Mice Overexpressing H2-Histamine Receptors in the Heart. *J Pharmacol Exp Ther.* 2020a Sep;374(3):479-488. doi: 10.1124/jpet.120.000063.

Gergs U, Kirchhefer U, Bergmann F, Künstler B, Mißlinger N, Au B, Mahnkopf M, Wache H, Neumann J (2020b) Characterization of stressed transgenic mice overexpressing H2-histamine-receptors. *J Pharmacol Exp Ther* 374:479–488. doi: 10.1124/jpet.120.000063.

Gergs U, Weisgut J, Griethe K, Mißlinger N, Kirchhefer U, Neumann J (2021) Human histamine H2 receptors can initiate cardiac arrhythmias in a transgenic mouse. *Naunyn-Schmiedeberg's Archives of Pharmacology* (in press).

Ginsburg R, Bristow MR, Davis K, Dibiase A, Billingham ME. Quantitative pharmacologic responses of normal and atherosclerotic isolated human epicardial coronary arteries. *Circulation.* 1984b Feb;69(2):430-40.

Ginsburg R, Bristow MR, Davis K. Receptor mechanisms in the human epicardial coronary artery. Heterogeneous pharmacological response to histamine and carbachol. *Circ Res.* 1984a Sep;55(3):416-21.

Ginsburg R, Bristow MR, Kantrowitz N, Baim DS, Harrison DC. Histamine provocation of clinical coronary artery spasm: implications concerning pathogenesis of variant angina pectoris. *Am Heart J.* 1981 Nov;102(5):819-22.

Ginsburg R, Bristow MR, Stinson EB, Harrison DC. Histamine receptors in the human heart. *Life Sci.* 1980 Jun 30;26(26):2245-9.

Giotti A, Guidotti A, Mannaioni PF, Zilletti L. The influences of andrenotropic drugs and noradrenaline on the histamine release in cardiac anaphylaxis in vitro. *J Physiol.* 1966 Jun;184(4):924-41.

Grange C, Gurrieri M, Verta R, Fantozzi R, Pini A, Rosa AC. Histamine in the kidneys: what is its role in renal pathophysiology? *Br J Pharmacol.* 2020 Feb;177(3):503-515. doi: 10.1111/bph.14619.

Grauers Wiktorin H, Nilsson MS, Kiffin R, Sander FE, Lenox B, Rydström A, Hellstrand K, Martner A. Histamine targets myeloid-derived suppressor cells and improves the anti-tumor efficacy of PD-1/PD-L1 checkpoint blockade. *Cancer Immunol Immunother.* 2019 Feb;68(2):163-174. doi: 10.1007/s00262-018-2253-6.

Grimsby J, Toth M, Chen K, Kumazawa T, Klaidman L, Adams JD, Karoum F, Gal J, Shih JC. Increased stress response and beta-phenylethylamine in MAOB-deficient mice. *Nat Genet.* 1997 Oct;17(2):206-10. doi: 10.1038/ng1097-206.

Gründemann D, Schechinger B, Rappold GA, Schömig E. Molecular identification of the corticosterone-sensitive extraneuronal catecholamine transporter. *Nat Neurosci.* 1998 Sep;1(5):349-51.

Hashikawa-Hobara N, Chan NY, Levi R. Histamine 3 receptor activation reduces the expression of neuronal angiotensin II type 1 receptors in the heart. *J Pharmacol Exp Ther.* 2012 Jan;340(1):185-91.

Hass C, Panda BP, Khanam R, Najmi AK, Akhtar M. Histamine H3 Receptor Agonist Imetit Attenuated Isoproterenol Induced Renin Angiotensin System and Sympathetic Nervous System Overactivity in Myocardial Infarction of

Rats. *Drug Res* (Stuttg). 2016 Jun;66(6):324-9. doi: 10.1055/s-0035-1569448.

Hatta E, Yasuda K, Levi R. Activation of histamine H3 receptors inhibits carrier-mediated norepinephrine release in a human model of protracted myocardial ischemia. *J Pharmacol Exp Ther.* 1997 Nov;283(2):494-500.

Hattori M, Yamazaki M, Ohashi W, Tanaka S, Hattori K, Todoroki K, Fujimori T, Ohtsu H, Matsuda N, Hattori Y. Critical role of endogenous histamine in promoting end-organ tissue injury in sepsis. *Intensive Care Med Exp.* 2016 Dec;4(1):36. doi: 10.1186/s40635-016-0109-y.

Hattori Y, Hattori K, Matsuda N. Regulation of the Cardiovascular System by Histamine. *Handb Exp Pharmacol.* 2017;241:239-258. doi: 10.1007/164_2016_15.

Hattori Y. Cardiac histamine receptors: their pharmacological consequences and signal transduction pathways. *Methods Find Exp Clin Pharmacol.* 1999 Mar;21(2):123-31. doi: 10.1358/mf.1999.21.2.529239.

He G, Hu J, Li T, Ma X, Meng J, Jia M, Lu J, Ohtsu H, Chen Z, Luo X. Arrhythmogenic effect of sympathetic histamine in mouse hearts subjected to acute ischemia. *Mol Med.* 2012 Feb 10;18:1-9.

He GH, Cai WK, Zhang JB, Ma CY, Yan F, Lu J, Xu GL. Associations of Polymorphisms in HRH2, HRH3, DAO, and HNMT Genes with Risk of Chronic Heart Failure. *Biomed Res Int.* 2016;2016:1208476.

Hescheler J, Tang M, Jastorff B, Trautwein W. On the mechanism of histamine induced enhancement of the cardiac Ca2+ current. *Pflugers Arch.* 1987 Sep;410(1-2):23-9.

Hirasawa N. Expression of Histidine Decarboxylase and Its Roles in Inflammation. *Int J Mol Sci.* 2019 Jan 16;20(2):376. doi: 10.3390/ijms20020376.

Höcker M, Rosenberg I, Xavier R, Henihan RJ, Wiedenmann B, Rosewicz S, Podolsky DK, Wang TC. Oxidative stress activates the human histidine decarboxylase promoter in AGS gastric cancer cells. *J Biol Chem.* 1998 Sep 4;273(36):23046-54. doi: 10.1074/jbc.273.36.23046.

Hofstra CL, Desai PJ, Thurmond RL, Fung-Leung WP Histamine H4 receptor mediates chemotaxis and calcium mobilization of mast cells. *J Pharmacol Exp Ther.* 2003 Jun;305(3):1212-21.

Houki S. Restoration effects of histamine on action potential in potassium-depolarized guinea-pig papillary muscle. *Arch Int Pharmacodyn Ther.* 1973 Nov;206(1):113-20.

Huang M, Pang X, Letourneau R, Boucher W, Theoharides TC. Acute stress induces cardiac mast cell activation and histamine release, effects that are increased in Apolipoprotein E knockout mice. *Cardiovasc Res.* 2002 Jul;55(1):150-60.

Humbert-Claude M, Davenas E, Gbahou F, Vincent L, Arrang JM. Involvement of histamine receptors in the atypical antipsychotic profile of clozapine: a reassessment in vitro and in vivo. *Psychopharmacology* (Berl). 2012 Mar;220(1):225-41. doi: 10.1007/s00213-011-2471-5.

Ichikawa A, Sugimoto Y, Tanaka S. Molecular biology of histidine decarboxylase and prostaglandin receptors. *Proc Jpn Acad Ser B Phys Biol Sci.* 2010;86(8):848-66. doi: 10.2183/pjab.86.848.

Imamura M, Lander HM, Levi R. Activation of histamine H3-receptors inhibits carrier-mediated norepinephrine release during protracted myocardial ischemia. Comparison with adenosine A1-receptors and alpha2-adrenoceptors. *Circ Res.* 1996 Mar;78(3):475-81. doi: 10.1161/01.res.78.3.475.

Imamura M, Poli E, Omoniyi AT, Levi R. Unmasking of activated histamine H3-receptors in myocardial ischemia: their role as regulators of exocytotic norepinephrine release. *J Pharmacol Exp Ther.* 1994 Dec;271(3):1259-66.

Imamura M, Seyedi N, Lander HM, Levi R. Functional identification of histamine H3-receptors in the human heart. *Circ Res.* 1995 Jul;77(1):206-10. doi: 10.1161/01.res.77.1.206.

Imanishi N, Nakayama T, Asano M, Yatsunami K, Tomita K, Ichikawa A. Induction of histidine decarboxylase by dexamethasone in mastocytoma P-815 cells. *Biochim Biophys Acta.* 1987 Apr 22;928(2):227-34. doi: 10.1016/0167-4889(87)90125-x.

Ind PW, Brown MJ, Lhoste FJ, Macquin I, Dollery CT. Concentration effect relationships of infused histamine in normal volunteers. *Agents Actions.* 1982 Apr;12(1-2):12-6.

Inoue I, Taniuchi I, Kitamura D, Jenkins NA, Gilbert DJ, Copeland NG, Watanabe T. Characteristics of the mouse genomic histamine H1 receptor gene. *Genomics.* 1996 Aug 15;36(1):178-81. doi: 10.1006/geno.1996.0441.

Jäger F, *Ein neuer, für die Praxis brauchbarer Sekaleersatz (Tenosin) Münchner Medizinische Wochenschrift* 1913a; 31: 1714-1715. [*A new, usable secale substitute (tenosin) Münchner Medizinische Wochenschrift*]

Jäger F, Versuche zur Verwendung des β-Imidazolyläthylamins in der Geburtshilfe. *Zentralblatt für Gynäkologie* 1913b; 8: 265-269. [Attempts to use β-imidazolylethylamine in obstetrics.]

Jones BL, Kearns GL. Histamine: new thoughts about a familiar mediator. *Clin Pharmacol Ther.* 2011 Feb;89(2):189-97.

Kaliner M, Sigler R, Summers R, Shelhamer JH. Effects of infused histamine: analysis of the effects of H-1 and H-2 histamine receptor antagonists on cardiovascular and pulmonary responses. *J Allergy Clin Immunol.* 1981 Nov;68(5):365-71.

Kaludercic N, Takimoto E, Nagayama T, Feng N, Lai EW, Bedja D, Chen K, Gabrielson KL, Blakely RD, Shih JC, Pacak K, Kass DA, Di Lisa F, Paolocci N. Monoamine oxidase A-mediated enhanced catabolism of norepinephrine contributes to adverse remodeling and pump failure in hearts with pressure overload. *Circ Res.* 2010 Jan 8;106(1):193-202.

Karlstedt K, Jin C, Panula P. Expression of histamine receptor genes Hrh3 and Hrh4 in rat brain endothelial cells. *Br J Pharmacol.* 2013 Sep;170(1):58-66. doi: 10.1111/bph.12173.

Kehrer E, Die motorischen Funktionen des Uterus und ihre Beeinflussung durch Wehenmittel. *Münchner Medizinische Wochenschrift* 1912; 33: 1831-1833. [The motor functions of the uterus and how they are influenced by contractions. *Munich Medical Weekly*]

Kehrer, E, Der überlebende Uterus als Testobjekt für die Wertigkeit der Mutterkorn-Präparate. *Archiv f. experiment. Pathol. u. Pharmakol* 58, 366–384 (1908). https://doi.org/10.1007/BF01841692.

Kitamura Y, Das AK, Murata Y, Maeyama K, Dev S, Wakayama Y, Kalubi B, Takeda N, Fukui H. Dexamethasone suppresses histamine synthesis by repressing both transcription and activity of HDC in allergic rats. *Allergol Int.* 2006 Sep;55(3):279-86. doi: 10.2332/allergolint.55.279.

Kitbunnadaj R, Zuiderveld OP, Christophe B, Hulscher S, Menge WM, Gelens E, Snip E, Bakker RA, Celanire S, Gillard M, Talaga P, Timmerman H, Leurs R. Identification of 4-(1H-imidazol-4(5)-ylmethyl)pyridine (immethridine) as a novel, potent, and highly selective histamine H(3) receptor agonist. *J Med Chem.* 2004 May 6;47(10):2414-7. doi: 10.1021/jm049932u.

Klocker J, Mätzler SA, Huetz GN, Drasche A, Kolbitsch C, Schwelberger HG. Expression of histamine degrading enzymes in porcine tissues. *Inflamm Res.* 2005 Apr;54 Suppl 1:S54-7.

Kobayashi T, Tonai S, Ishihara Y, Koga R, Okabe S, Watanabe T. Abnormal functional and morphological regulation of the gastric mucosa in histamine H2 receptor-deficient mice. *J Clin Invest.* 2000 Jun;105(12):1741-9.

Kolosova IA, Ma SF, Adyshev DM, Wang P, Ohba M, Natarajan V, Garcia JG, Verin AD. Role of CPI-17 in the regulation of endothelial cytoskeleton. *Am J Physiol Lung Cell Mol Physiol.* 2004 Nov;287(5):L970-80. doi: 10.1152/ajplung.00398.2003.

Kounis NG, Koniari I, Tzanis G, Soufras GD, Velissaris D, Hahalis G. Anaphylaxis-induced atrial fibrillation and anesthesia: Pathophysiologic and therapeutic considerations. *Ann Card Anaesth.* 2020 Jan-Mar;23(1):1-6. doi: 10.4103/aca.ACA_100_19.

Koyama M, Heerdt PM, Levi R. Increased severity of reperfusion arrhythmias in mouse hearts lacking histamine H3-receptors. *Biochem Biophys Res Commun.* 2003a Jul 4;306(3):792-6.

Koyama M, Seyedi N, Fung-Leung WP, Lovenberg TW, Levi R. Norepinephrine release from the ischemic heart is greatly enhanced in mice lacking histamine H3 receptors. *Mol Pharmacol.* 2003b Feb;63(2):378-82.

Kritikou E, Kuiper J, Kovanen PT, Bot I. The impact of mast cells on cardiovascular diseases. *Eur J Pharmacol.* 2016 May 5;778:103-15.

Laher I, McNeill JH. Effects of histamine in the isolated kitten heart. *Can J Physiol Pharmacol.* 1980c Nov;58(11):1256-61.

Laher I, McNeill JH. Effects of histamine on rat isolated atria. *Can J Physiol Pharmacol.* 1980a Sep;58(9):1114-6.

Lai TS, Greenberg CS. Histaminylation of fibrinogen by tissue transglutaminase-2 (TGM-2): potential role in modulating inflammation. *Amino Acids.* 2013 Oct;45(4):857-64.

Lai X, Ye L, Liao Y, Jin L, Ma Q, Lu B, Sun Y, Shi Y, Zhou N. Agonist-induced activation of histamine H3 receptor signals to extracellular signal-regulated kinases 1 and 2 through PKC-, PLD-, and EGFR-dependent mechanisms. *J Neurochem.* 2016 Apr;137(2):200-15. doi: 10.1111/jnc.13559.

Laroche D, Dubois F, Gérard JL, Lefrançois C, André B, Vergnaud MC, Dubus L, Bricard H. Radioimmunoassay for plasma histamine: a study of false positive and false negative values. *Br J Anaesth.* 1995 Apr;74(4):430-7.

Layritz CM, Hagel AF, Graf V, Reiser C, Klinghammer L, Ropers D, Achenbach S, Raithel M. Histamine in atrial fibrillation (AF)--is there any connection? Results from an unselected population. *Int J Cardiol.* 2014 Apr 1;172(3):e432-3.

Leary PJ, Kronmal RA, Bluemke DA, Buttrick PM, Jones KL, Kao DP, Kawut SM, Krieger EV, Lima JA, Minobe W, Ralph DD, Tedford RJ, Weiss NS, Bristow MR. Histamine H2 Receptor Polymorphisms, Myocardial Transcripts, and Heart Failure (from the Multi-Ethnic Study of Atherosclerosis and Beta-Blocker Effect on Remodeling and Gene Expression Trial). *Am J Cardiol.* 2018 Jan 15;121(2):256-261.

Ledda F, Mugelli A, Mantelli L. A histamine-induced decrease of action potential duration in cardiac muscle mediated by the H2 receptors. *Agents Actions.* 1977 Jul;7(2):199-202. doi: 10.1007/BF01969972.

Levi R and Allan G (1980) Histamine-mediated cardiac effects. In: Bristow M (ed.) *Drug-induced and heart disease.* Elsevier /North Holland, Amsterdam. Pp377-395.

Levi R, Capurro N, Lee CH. Pharmacological characterization of cardiac histamine receptors: sensitivity to H1-and H2-receptor agonists and antagonists. *Eur J Pharmacol.* 1975 Feb;30(2):328-35.

Levi R, Kuye JO. Pharmacological characterization of cardiac histamine receptors: sensitivity to H1-receptor antagonists. *Eur J Pharmacol.* 1974 Aug;27(3):330-8.

Levi R, Pappano AJ. Modification of the effects of histamine and norepinephrine on the sinoatrial node pacemaker by potassium and calcium. *J Pharmacol Exp Ther.* 1978 Mar;204(3):625-33.

Levi R, Rubin LE, Gross SS (1991) histamine in cardiovascular function and dysfunction: recent developments. In: Uvnäs B (ed.) Handbook of experimental pharmacology. *Histamine and histamine antagonists,* vol 97. Springer, Berlin, pp 347-383.

Levi R, Seyedi N, Schaefer U, Estephan R, Mackins CJ, Tyler E, Silver RB. Histamine H3-receptor signaling in cardiac sympathetic nerves: Identification of a novel MAPK-PLA2-COX-PGE2-EP3R pathway. *Biochem Pharmacol.* 2007 Apr 15;73(8):1146-56.

Levi R, Smith NC. Histamine H(3)-receptors: a new frontier in myocardial ischemia. *J Pharmacol Exp Ther.* 2000 Mar;292(3):825-30.

Levi R. Effects of exogenous and immunologically released histamine on the isolated heart: a quantitative comparison. *J Pharmacol Exp Ther.* 1972 Aug;182(2):227-38.

Levick SP, Gardner JD, Holland M, Hauer-Jensen M, Janicki JS, Brower GL. Protection from adverse myocardial remodeling secondary to chronic volume overload in mast cell deficient rats. *J Mol Cell Cardiol.* 2008 Jul;45(1):56-61.

Levick SP, Meléndez GC, Plante E, McLarty JL, Brower GL, Janicki JS. Cardiac mast cells: the centrepiece in adverse myocardial remodelling. *Cardiovasc Res.* 2011 Jan 1;89(1):12-9.

Levine RJ, Sato TL, Sjoerdsma A. Inhibiton of histamine sysnthesein in the rat by alpha-hydrazino analog of histidine and 4-bromo-3-hydyroxy benzyloxyamine. *Biochem Pharmacol.* 1965 Feb;14:139-49.

Li H, Burkhardt C, Heinrich UR, Brausch I, Xia N, Förstermann U. Histamine upregulates gene expression of endothelial nitric oxide synthase in human vascular endothelial cells. *Circulation.* 2003 May 13;107(18):2348-54.

Li M, Hu J, Chen Z, Meng J, Wang H, Ma X, Luo X. Evidence for histamine as a neurotransmitter in the cardiac sympathetic nervous system. *Am J Physiol Heart Circ Physiol.* 2006 Jul;291(1):H45-51. doi: 10.1152/ajpheart. 00939.2005.

Li X, Eschun G, Bose D, Jacobs H, Yang JJ, Light RB, Mink SN. Histamine H3 activation depresses cardiac function in experimental sepsis. *J Appl Physiol (1985).* 1998 Nov;85(5):1693-701.

Liao CH, Akazawa H, Tamagawa M, Ito K, Yasuda N, Kudo Y, Yamamoto R, Ozasa Y, Fujimoto M, Wang P, Nakauchi H, Nakaya H, Komuro I. Cardiac mast cells cause atrial fibrillation through PDGF-A-mediated fibrosis in pressure-overloaded mouse hearts. *J Clin Invest.* 2010 Jan;120(1):242-53. doi: 10.1172/JCI39942.

Lin RY, Schwartz LB, Curry A, Pesola GR, Knight RJ, Lee HS, Bakalchuk L, Tenenbaum C, Westfal RE. Histamine and tryptase levels in patients with acute allergic reactions: An emergency department-based study. *J Allergy Clin Immunol.* 2000 Jul;106(1 Pt 1):65-71. doi: 10.1067/mai.2000.107600.

Lindell Se, Nilsson K, Roos Be, Westling H. The effect of enzyme inhibitors on histamine catabolism in man. *Br J Pharmacol Chemother.* 1960 Jun;15(2):351-5. doi: 10.1111/j.1476-5381.1960.tb01255.x.

Llenas J, Cardelús I, Heredia A, de Mora F, Gristwood RW. Cardiotoxicity of histamine and the possible role of histamine in the arrhythmogenesis produced by certain antihistamines. *Drug Saf.* 1999;21 Suppl 1:33-8; discussion 81-7. doi: 10.2165/00002018-199921001-00005.

Lorenz W, Gerant M, Werle E. Induction of the specific histidine decarboxylase by TSH and 2-mercaptobenzimidazole-1,3-dimethylol (MBI). *Naunyn Schmiedebergs Arch Exp Pathol Pharmakol.* 1968;260(2):171-2. doi: 10.1007/BF00537981.

Luo T, Chen B, Zhao Z, He N, Zeng Z, Wu B, Fukushima Y, Dai M, Huang Q, Xu D, Bin J, Kitakaze M, Liao Y. Histamine H2 receptor activation exacerbates myocardial ischemia/reperfusion injury by disturbing mitochondrial and endothelial function. *Basic Res Cardiol.* 2013 May;108(3):342.

Luo XX, Tan YH, Sheng BH. Histamine H3-receptors inhibit sympathetic neurotransmission in guinea pig myocardium. *Eur J Pharmacol.* 1991 Nov 12;204(3):311-4.

Mackins CJ, Kano S, Seyedi N, Schäfer U, Reid AC, Machida T, Silver RB, Levi R. Cardiac mast cell-derived renin promotes local angiotensin formation, norepinephrine release, and arrhythmias in ischemia/reperfusion. *J Clin Invest.* 2006 Apr;116(4):1063-70. doi: 10.1172/JCI25713.

Maintz L, Bieber T, Novak N. Die verschiedenen Gesicher der Histaminintoleranz. *Deutsches Ärzteblatt* 2006;103 (51-52):B3027-B3033.

Maintz L, Novak N. Histamine and histamine intolerance. *Am J Clin Nutr.* 2007 May;85(5):1185-96.

Maltsev AV, Kokoz YM, Evdokimovskii EV, Pimenov OY, Reyes S, Alekseev AE. Alpha-2 adrenoceptors and imidazoline receptors in cardiomyocytes mediate counterbalancing effect of agmatine on NO synthesis and intracellular calcium handling. *J Mol Cell Cardiol.* 2014 Mar;68:66-74.

Martinel Lamas DJ, Nicoud MB, Sterle HA, Carabajal E, Tesan F, Perazzo JC, Cremaschi GA, Rivera ES, Medina VA. Selective cytoprotective effect of histamine on doxorubicin-induced hepatic and cardiac toxicity in animal models. *Cell Death Discov.* 2015 Dec 21;1:15059. doi: 10.1038/cddiscovery.2015.59.

Masini E, Bianchi S, Mugnai L, Gambassi F, Lupini M, Pistelli A, Mannaioni PF. The effect of nitric oxide generators on ischemia reperfusion injury and histamine release in isolated perfused guinea-pig heart. *Agents Actions.* 1991 May;33(1-2):53-6.

Masini E, Phanchenault J, Pezziardi F, Gautier P, Gagnol JP. Histamine release during an experimental coronary thrombosis in awake dog. *Agents Actions.* 1985 Apr;16(3-4):227-30. doi: 10.1007/BF01983146.

Masini E, Vannacci A, Marzocca C, Mannaioni PF, Befani O, Federico R, Toma A, Mondovì B. A plant histaminase modulates cardiac anaphylactic response in guinea pig. *Biochem Biophys Res Commun.* 2002 Aug 30;296(4):840-6. doi: 10.1016/s0006-291x(02)00938-5.

Matsuda N, Hattori Y, Sakuraya F, Kobayashi M, Zhang XH, Kemmotsu O, Gando S. Hemodynamic significance of histamine synthesis and histamine H1- and H2-receptor gene expression during endotoxemia. *Naunyn Schmiedebergs Arch Pharmacol.* 2002 Dec;366(6):513-21.

Matsuda N, Jesmin S, Takahashi Y, Hatta E, Kobayashi M, Matsuyama K, Kawakami N, Sakuma I, Gando S, Fukui H, Hattori Y, Levi R. Histamine H1 and H2 receptor gene and protein levels are differentially expressed in the hearts of rodents and humans. *J Pharmacol Exp Ther.* 2004 May;309(2):786-95. doi: 10.1124/jpet.103.063065.

Mazenot C, Durand A, Ribuot C, Demenge P, Godin-Ribuot D. Histamine H3-receptor stimulation is unable to modulate noradrenaline release by the isolated rat heart during ischaemia-reperfusion. *Fundam Clin Pharmacol.* 1999b;13(4):455-60. doi: 10.1111/j.1472-8206.1999.tb00003.x.

Mazenot C, Ribuot C, Durand A, Joulin Y, Demenge P, Godin-Ribuot D. In vivo demonstration of H3-histaminergic inhibition of cardiac sympathetic stimulation by R-alpha-methyl-histamine and its prodrug BP 2.94 in the dog. *Br J Pharmacol.* 1999a Jan;126(1):264-8. doi: 10.1038/sj.bjp.0702257.

McCaffrey SL, Lim G, Bullock M, Kasparian AO, Clifton-Bligh R, Campbell WB, Widiapradja A, Levick SP. The Histamine 3 Receptor Is Expressed in the Heart and Its Activation Opposes Adverse Cardiac Remodeling in the Angiotensin II Mouse Model. *Int J Mol Sci.* 2020 Dec 21;21(24):9757. doi: 10.3390/ijms21249757.

McGrath AP, Hilmer KM, Collyer CA, Dooley DM, Guss JM. new crystal form of human diamine oxidase. *Acta Crystallogr Sect F Struct Biol Cryst Commun.* 2010 Feb 1;66(Pt 2):137-42.

McNeil JH histamine and the heart. *Can J Physiol Pharmacol* 126: 264-268.

Miura Y, Yoshikawa T, Naganuma F, Nakamura T, Iida T, Kárpáti A, Matsuzawa T, Mogi A, Harada R, Yanai K. Characterization of murine polyspecific monoamine transporters. *FEBS Open Bio.* 2017 Jan 9;7(2):237-248.

Moore JN, Drury MO. Antabus in the management of chronic alcoholism. *Lancet.* 1951 Dec 8;2(6693):1059-61. doi: 10.1016/s0140-6736(51)92976-5.

Moore TC, Chang JK. Urinary histamine excretion in the rat following skin homografting and autografting. *Ann Surg.* 1968 Feb;167(2):232-8.

Moreno-Delgado D, Puigdellívol M, Moreno E, Rodríguez-Ruiz M, Botta J, Gasperini P, Chiarlone A, Howell LA, Scarselli M, Casadó V, Cortés A, Ferré S, Guzmán M, Lluís C, Alberch J, Canela EI, Ginés S, McCormick PJ. Modulation of dopamine D1 receptors via histamine H3 receptors is a novel therapeutic target for Huntington's disease. *Elife.* 2020 Jun 9;9:e51093. doi: 10.7554/eLife.51093.

Moriguchi T, Takai J. Histamine and histidine decarboxylase: Immunomodulatory functions and regulatory mechanisms. *Genes Cells.* 2020 Jul;25(7):443-449. doi: 10.1111/gtc.12774.

Morrow JD, Margolies GR, Rowland J, Roberts LJ 2nd. Evidence that histamine is the causative toxin of scombroid-fish poisoning. *N Engl J Med.* 1991 Mar 14;324(11):716-20. doi: 10.1056/NEJM199103143241102.

Moss J, De Mello MC, Vaughan M, Beaven MA. Effect of salicylates on histamine and L-histidine metabolism. Inhibition of imidazoleacetate phosphoribosyl transferase. *J Clin Invest.* 1976 Jul;58(1):137-41. doi: 10.1172/JCI108442.

Naganuma F, Yoshikawa T, Nakamura T, Iida T, Harada R, Mohsen AS, Miura Y, Yanai K. Predominant role of plasma membrane monoamine transporters in monoamine transport in 1321N1, a human astrocytoma-derived cell line. *J Neurochem.* 2014 May;129(4):591-601.

Neugebauer E, Rixen D, Garcia-Caballero M, Scheid B, Lorenz W. Time sequence of histamine release and formation in rat endotoxic shock. *Shock.* 1994 Apr;1(4):299-306. doi: 10.1097/00024382-199404000-00009.

Neumann J, Binter MBB, Fehse C, Marusakova M, Kirchhefer U, Wache H, Hofmann B, Gergs U (2021c) Amitryptiline functionally antagonizes H2 receptors in transgenic mice and human atria. *Naunyn-Schmiedeberg's Archives of Pharmacology* doi: 10.1007/s00210-021-02065-7.

Neumann J, Grobe JM, Weisgut J, Schwelberger HG, Fogel WA, Marušáková M, Wache H, Bähre H, Buchwalow IB, Dhein S, Hofmann B, Kirchhefer U, Gergs U. Histamine can be Formed and Degraded in the Human and Mouse Heart. *Front Pharmacol.* 2021a May 11;12:582916. doi: 10.3389/fphar.2021.582916. *eCollection* 2021.

Neumann J, Voss R, Laufs U, Werner C, Gergs U (2021b) Phosphodiesterases 2, 3 and 4 can decrease cardiac effects of H2-histamine-receptor activation in isolated atria of transgenic mice. *Naunyn-Schmiedeberg's Archives of Pharmacology* doi: 10.1007/s00210-021-02052-y.

Niijima-Yaoita F, Tsuchiya M, Ohtsu H, Yanai K, Sugawara S, Endo Y, Tadano T. Roles of histamine in exercise-induced fatigue: favouring endurance and protecting against exhaustion. *Biol Pharm Bull.* 2012;35(1):91-7. doi: 10.1248/bpb.35.91.

Noguchi K, Ishida J, Kim JD, Muromachi N, Kako K, Mizukami H, Lu W, Ishimaru T, Kawasaki S, Kaneko S, Usui J, Ohtsu H, Yamagata K, Fukamizu A. Histamine receptor agonist alleviates severe cardiorenal damages by eliciting anti-inflammatory programming. *Proc Natl Acad Sci U S A.* 2020 Feb 11;117(6):3150-3156. doi: 10.1073/pnas.1909124117.

Ogasawara M, Yamauchi K, Satoh Y, Yamaji R, Inui K, Jonker JW, Schinkel AH, Maeyama K. Recent advances in molecular pharmacology of the histamine systems: organic cation transporters as a histamine transporter and histamine metabolism. *J Pharmacol Sci.* 2006 May;101(1):24-30. doi: 10.1254/jphs. fmj06001x6.

Ohtsu H, Tanaka S, Terui T, Hori Y, Makabe-Kobayashi Y, Pejler G, Tchougounova E, Hellman L, Gertsenstein M, Hirasawa N, Sakurai E, Buzás E, Kovács P, Csaba G, Kittel A, Okada M, Hara M, Mar L, Numayama-Tsuruta K, Ishigaki-Suzuki S, Ohuchi K, Ichikawa A, Falus A, Watanabe T, Nagy A. Mice lacking histidine decarboxylase exhibit abnormal mast cells. *FEBS Lett.* 2001 Jul 27;502(1-2):53-6. doi: 10.1016/s0014-5793(01)02663-1.

Ohtsu H. Progress in allergy signal research on mast cells: the role of histamine in immunological and cardiovascular disease and the transporting system of histamine in the cell. *J Pharmacol Sci.* 2008 Mar;106(3):347-53. doi: 10.1254/jphs.fm0070294.

Ohtsubo T, Rovira II, Starost MF, Liu C, Finkel T. Xanthine oxidoreductase is an endogenous regulator of cyclooxygenase-2. *Circ Res.* 2004 Nov 26;95(11):1118-24. doi: 10.1161/01.RES.0000149571.96304.36.

Oyama T, Isse T, Kagawa N, Kinaga T, Kim YD, Morita M, Sugio K, Weiner H, Yasumoto K, Kawamoto T. Tissue-distribution of aldehyde dehydrogenase 2 and effects of the ALDH2 gene-disruption on the expression of enzymes involved in alcohol metabolism. *Front Biosci.* 2005 Jan 1;10:951-60. doi: 10.2741/1589.

Ozono R, O'Connell DP, Wang ZQ, Moore AF, Sanada H, Felder RA, Carey RM. Localization of the dopamine D1 receptor protein in the human heart and kidney. *Hypertension.* 1997 Sep;30(3 Pt 2):725-9.

Panula P, Chazot PL, Cowart M, Gutzmer R, Leurs R, Liu WL, Stark H, Thurmond RL, Haas HL International Union of Basic and Clinical Pharmacology. XCVIII. Histamine Receptors. *Pharmacol Rev.* 2015 Jul;67(3):601-55.

Patella V, Marinò I, Arbustini E, Lamparter-Schummert B, Verga L, Adt M, Marone G. Stem cell factor in mast cells and increased mast cell density in idiopathic and ischemic cardiomyopathy. *Circulation.* 1998 Mar 17;97(10):971-8.

Penna M, Illanes A, Ubilla M, Mujica S. Effect of histamine and of The anaphylactic reaction on isolated guinea pig atria. *Circ Res.* 1959 Jul;7(4):521-6.

Perin A, Sessa A, Desiderio MA. Polyamine levels and diamine oxidase activity in hypertrophic heart of spontaneously hypertensive rats and of rats treated with isoproterenol. *Biochim Biophys Acta.* 1983 Feb 22;755(3):344-51. doi: 10.1016/0304-4165(83)90236-2.

Piera L, Olczak S, Kun T, Galdyszynska M, Ciosek J, Szymanski J, Drobnik J. Disruption of histamine/H3 receptor signal reduces collagen deposition in cultures scar myofibroblasts. *J Physiol Pharmacol.* 2019 Apr;70(2). doi: 10.26402/jpp.2019.2.07.

Pierpaoli S, Marzocca C, Bello MG, Schunack W, Mannaioni PF, Masini E. Histaminergic receptors modulate the coronary vascular response in isolated guinea pig hearts. Role of nitric oxide. *Inflamm Res.* 2003 Sep;52(9):390-6.

Plapp BV, Leidal KG, Smith RK, Murch BP. Kinetics of inhibition of ethanol metabolism in rats and the rate-limiting role of alcohol dehydrogenase. *Arch Biochem Biophys.* 1984 Apr;230(1):30-8. doi: 10.1016/0003-9861(84)90083-3.

Preuss H, Ghorai P, Kraus A, Dove S, Buschauer A, Seifert R. Mutations of Cys-17 and Ala-271 in the human histamine H2 receptor determine the species selectivity of guanidine-type agonists and increase constitutive activity. *J Pharmacol Exp Ther.* 2007 Jun;321(3):975-82.

Pugin B, Barcik W, Westermann P, Heider A, Wawrzyniak M, Hellings P, Akdis CA, O'Mahony L. A wide diversity of bacteria from the human gut produces and degrades biogenic amines. *Microb Ecol Health Dis.* 2017 Jan 1;28(1):1353881. doi: 10.1080/16512235.2017.1353881.

Reid AC, Brazin JA, Morrey C, Silver RB, Levi R. Targeting cardiac mast cells: pharmacological modulation of the local renin-angiotensin system. *Curr Pharm Des.* 2011 Nov;17(34):3744-52.

Renz CL, Laroche D, Thurn JD, Finn HA, Lynch JP, Thisted R, Moss J. Tryptase levels are not increased during vancomycin-induced anaphylactoid reactions. *Anesthesiology.* 1998 Sep;89(3):620-5. doi: 10.1097/00000542-199809000-00010.

Riley JF. Histamine and Sir Henry Dale Dale. *Br Med J.* 1965 Jun 5;1(5448):1488–1490.

Rioux F, Kérouac R, St-Pierre S. Neurotensin stimulates histamine release from the isolated, spontaneously beating heart of rats. *Life Sci.* 1984 Jul 23;35(4):423-31.

Rohr SM, Rich MW, Silver KH. Shortness of breath, syncope, and cardiac arrest caused by systemic mastocytosis. *Ann Emerg Med.* 2005 Jun;45(6):592-4.

Rojas-Perez-Ezquerra P, Noguerado-Mellado B, Morales-Cabeza C, Zambrano Ibarra G, Datino Romaniega T. Atrial Fibrillation in Anaphylaxis. *Am J Med.* 2017 Sep;130(9):1114-1116.

Sanders L, Lynham JA, Kaumann AJ. Chronic beta 1-adrenoceptor blockade sensitises the H1 and H2 receptor systems in human atrium: role of cyclic nucleotides. *Naunyn Schmiedebergs Arch Pharmacol.* 1996 May;353(6):661-70.

Schenk P. Über die Wirkungsweise des β-Imidazoläthylamins (Histamins) auf den menschlichen Organismus. *Arch exp Pathol Pharmacol* 1921; 89:332-339. About the mode of action of β-imidazolethylamine (histamine) on the human organism. *Arch exp Pathol Pharmacol*]

Schirone M, Visciano P, Tofalo R, Suzzi G. Histamine Food Poisoning. *Handb Exp Pharmacol.* 2017;241:217-235. doi: 10.1007/164_2016_54.

Schoenwald PK, Sprung J, Abdelmalak B, Mraović B, Tetzlaff JE, Gurm HS. Complete atrioventricular block and cardiac arrest following intravenous famotidine administration. *Anesthesiology.* 1999 Feb;90(2):623-6.

Schwelberger HG, Feurle J, Ahrens F. Characterization of diamine oxidase from human seminal plasma. *J Neural Transm* (Vienna). 2013 Jun;120(6):983-6. doi: 10.1007/s00702-013-0983-3.

Schwelberger HG, Feurle J, Houen G. Mapping of the binding sites of human diamine oxidase (DAO) monoclonal antibodies. *Inflamm Res.* 2018 Mar;67(3):245-253. doi: 10.1007/s00011-017-1118-3.

Seifert R, Strasser A, Schneider EH, Neumann D, Dove S, Buschauer A. Molecular and cellular analysis of human histamine receptor subtypes. *Trends Pharmacol Sci.* 2013 Jan;34(1):33-58.

Senges J, Randolf U, Katus H. Ventricular arrhythmias in cardiac anaphylaxis. *Naunyn Schmiedebergs Arch Pharmacol.* 1977 Nov;300(2):115-21.

Sessa A, Perin A. Diamine oxidase in relation to diamine and polyamine metabolism. *Agents Actions.* 1994 Nov;43(1-2):69-77. doi: 10.1007/BF02005768.

Seyedi N, Mackins CJ, Machida T, Reid AC, Silver RB, Levi R. Histamine H3-receptor-induced attenuation of norepinephrine exocytosis: a decreased protein kinase a activity mediates a reduction in intracellular calcium. *J Pharmacol Exp Ther.* 2005 Jan;312(1):272-80. doi: 10.1124/jpet.104.072504.

Seyedi N, Maruyama R, Levi R. Bradykinin activates a cross-signaling pathway between sensory and adrenergic nerve endings in the heart: a novel mechanism of ischemic norepinephrine release? *J Pharmacol Exp Ther.* 1999 Aug;290(2):656-63.

Shaffer HC, Parsons DJ, Peden DB, Morrell D Recurrent syncope and anaphylaxis as presentation of systemic mastocytosis in a pediatric patient: case report and literature review. *J Am Acad Dermatol.* 2006 May;54(5 Suppl):S210-3.

Shimokawa H, Tomoike H, Nabeyama S, Yamamoto H, Araki H, Nakamura M, Ishii Y, Tanaka K. Coronary artery spasm induced in atherosclerotic miniature swine. *Science.* 1983 Aug 5;221(4610):560-2.

Simons FE, Simons KJ. Histamine and H1-antihistamines: celebrating a century of progress. *J Allergy Clin Immunol.* 2011 Dec;128(6):1139-1150.

Stegaev V, Nies AT, Porola P, Mieliauskaite D, Sánchez-Jiménez F, Urdiales JL, Sillat T, Schwelberger HG, Chazot PL, Katebe M, Mackiewicz Z, Konttinen YT, Nordström DC. Histamine transport and metabolism are deranged in salivary glands in Sjogren's syndrome. *Rheumatology* (Oxford). 2013 Sep;52(9):1599-608.

Stolen CM, Marttila-Ichihara F, Koskinen K, Yegutkin GG, Turja R, Bono P, Skurnik M, Hänninen A, Jalkanen S, Salmi M. Absence of the endothelial oxidase AOC3 leads to abnormal leukocyte traffic in vivo. *Immunity.* 2005 Jan;22(1):105-15.

Stolen CM, Yegutkin GG, Kurkijärvi R, Bono P, Alitalo K, Jalkanen S. Origins of serum semicarbazide-sensitive amine oxidase. *Circ Res.* 2004 Jul 9;95(1):50-7.

Takahashi K, Suwa H, Ishikawa T, Kotani H. Targeted disruption of H3 receptors results in changes in brain histamine tone leading to an obese phenotype. *J Clin Invest.* 2002 Dec;110(12):1791-9. doi: 10.1172/JCI15784.

Takai J, Ohtsu H, Sato A, Uemura S, Fujimura T, Yamamoto M, Moriguchi T. Lipopolysaccharide-induced expansion of histidine decarboxylase-expressing Ly6G+ myeloid cells identified by exploiting histidine decarboxylase BAC-GFP transgenic mice. *Sci Rep.* 2019 Oct 30;9(1):15603. doi: 10.1038/s41598-019-51716-6.

Tan X, Essengue S, Talreja J, Reese J, Stechschulte DJ, Dileepan KN. Histamine directly and synergistically with lipopolysaccharide stimulates cyclooxygenase-2 expression and prostaglandin I(2) and E(2) production in human coronary artery endothelial cells. *J Immunol.* 2007 Dec 1;179(11):7899-906.

Tanaka H, Furukawa T, Hayafuji M, Habuchi Y. Modulation of the delayed K+ current by histamine in guinea pig ventricular myocytes. Naunyn Schmiedebergs *Arch Pharmacol.* 1991 Nov;344(5):582-8. doi: 10.1007/BF00170656.

Tanaka H, Uesato N, Shigenobu K. Chronotropic and inotropic effects of histamine in developing chick heart: differential mechanisms before and after hatching. *Naunyn Schmiedebergs Arch Pharmacol.* 1995 Apr;351(4):391-7.

Taylor SL, Stratton JE, Nordlee JA. Histamine poisoning (scombroid fish poisoning): an allergy-like intoxication. *J Toxicol Clin Toxicol.* 1989;27(4-5):225-40.

Thangam EB, Jemima EA, Singh H, Baig MS, Khan M, Mathias CB, Church MK, Saluja R. The Role of Histamine and Histamine Receptors in Mast Cell-Mediated Allergy and Inflammation: The Hunt for New Therapeutic Targets. *Front Immunol.* 2018 Aug 13;9:1873. doi: 10.3389/fimmu.2018.01873.

Thoren FB, Aurelius J, Martner A. Antitumor properties of histamine in vivo. *Nat Med.* 2011 May;17(5):537.

Tiligada E, Ennis M. Histamine pharmacology: from Sir Henry Dale to the 21st century. *Br J Pharmacol.* 2020 Feb;177(3):469-489. doi: 10.1111/bph.14524.

Toyota H, Sugimoto N, Kobayashi K, Suzuki Y, Takeshita Y, Ito A, Ujino M, Tomyo F, Sakasegawa H, Koizumi Y, Kuramochi M, Yamaguchi M, Nagase H. Comprehensive analysis of allergen-specific IgE in COPD: mite-specific IgE specifically related to the diagnosis of asthma-COPD overlap. *Allergy Asthma Clin Immunol.* 2021 Feb 4;17(1):13. doi: 10.1186/s13223-021-00514-9.

Travis ER, Wang YM, Michael DJ, Caron MG, Wightman RM. Differential quantal release of histamine and 5-hydroxytryptamine from mast cells of vesicular monoamine transporter 2 knockout mice. *Proc Natl Acad Sci U S A.* 2000 Jan 4;97(1):162-7.

Tuck CJ, Biesiekierski JR, Schmid-Grendelmeier P, Pohl D. Food Intolerances. *Nutrients.* 2019 Jul 22;11(7):1684. doi: 10.3390/nu11071684.

Valen G, Kaszaki J, Nagy S, Vaage J. Open heart surgery increases the levels of histamine in arterial and coronary sinus blood. *Agents Actions.* 1994b Mar;41(1-2):11-6. doi: 10.1007/BF01986386.

Valen G, Kaszaki J, Szabo I, Nagy S, Vaage J. Histamine release and its effects in ischaemia-reperfusion injury of the isolated rat heart. *Acta Physiol Scand.* 1994 Apr;150(4):413-24. doi: 10.1111/j.1748-1716.1994.tb09706.x.

van der Linden PW, Hack CE, Poortman J, Vivié-Kipp YC, Struyvenberg A, van der Zwan JK. Insect-sting challenge in 138 patients: relation between clinical severity of anaphylaxis and mast cell activation. *J Allergy Clin Immunol.* 1992 Jul;90(1):110-8. doi: 10.1016/s0091-6749(06)80017-5.

Vigorito C, Russo P, Picotti GB, Chiariello M, Poto S, Marone G. Cardiovascular effects of histamine infusion in man. *J Cardiovasc Pharmacol.* 1983 Jul-Aug;5(4):531-7.

Villeneuve C, Guilbeau-Frugier C, Sicard P, Lairez O, Ordener C, Duparc T, De Paulis D, Couderc B, Spreux-Varoquaux O, Tortosa F, Garnier A, Knauf C,

Valet P, Borchi E, Nediani C, Gharib A, Ovize M, Delisle MB, Parini A, Mialet-Perez J. p53-PGC-1α pathway mediates oxidative mitochondrial damage and cardiomyocyte necrosis induced by monoamine oxidase-A upregulation: role in chronic left ventricular dysfunction in mice. *Antioxid Redox Signal.* 2013 Jan 1;18(1):5-18.

Walker AK, Park WM, Chuang JC, Perello M, Sakata I, Osborne-Lawrence S, Zigman JM. Characterization of gastric and neuronal histaminergic populations using a transgenic mouse model. *PLoS One.* 2013;8(3):e60276. doi: 10.1371/journal.pone.0060276.

Wansa N, Goethals P, DeRoy L. Histamine, paroxysmal AV block and low adenosine syncope a case report. *J Electrocardiol.* 2018 Jan-Feb;51(1):150-152. doi: 10.1016/j.jelectrocard.2017.09.003.

Wantke F, Hemmer W, Focke M, Haglmüller T, Götz M, Jarisch R. The red wine maximization test: drinking histamine rich wine induces a transient increase in plasma diamine oxidase activity in healthy volunteers. *Inflamm Res.* 1999 Apr;48(4):169-70. doi: 10.1007/s000110050441.

Wantke F, Proud D, Siekierski E, Kagey-Sobotka A. Daily variations of serum diamine oxidase and the influence of H1 and H2 blockers: a critical approach to routine diamine oxidase assessment. *Inflamm Res.* 1998 Oct;47(10):396-400.

Warren K, Dyer J, Merlin S, Kaliner M. Measurement of urinary histamine: comparison of fluorometric and radioisotopic-enzymatic assay procedures. *J Allergy Clin Immunol.* 1983 Feb;71(2):206-11. doi: 10.1016/0091-6749(83)90101-x. PMID: 6401774.

Werle E: Über die Bildung von Histamin aus Histidin durch tierisches Gewebe (1936). *Biochem Z.* 288:292-293. [About the formation of histamine from histidine by animal tissue]

Wolff AA, Levi R. Histamine and cardiac arrhythmias. *Circ Res.* 1986 Jan;58(1):1-16.

Yamada Y, Yoshikawa T, Naganuma F, Kikkawa T, Osumi N, Yanai K. Chronic brain histamine depletion in adult mice induced depression-like behaviours and impaired sleep-wake cycle. *Neuropharmacology.* 2020 Sep 15;175:108179. doi: 10.1016/j.neuropharm.2020.108179.

Yang LP, Perry CM. Histamine dihydrochloride: in the management of acute myeloid leukaemia. *Drugs.* 2011 Jan 1;71(1):109-22.

Yang XD, Ai W, Asfaha S, Bhagat G, Friedman RA, Jin GC, Park H, Shykind B, Diacovo TG, Falus A, Wang TC (2011) Histamine deficiency promotes inflammation-associated carcinogenesis through reduced myeloid maturation and accumulation of CD11b(+)Ly6G(+) immature myeloid cells. *Nat Med* 17(1):87–263.

Yokoyama A, Mori S, Takahashi HK, Kanke T, Wake H, Nishibori M. Effect of amodiaquine, a histamine N-methyltransferase inhibitor, on, Propionibacterium acnes and lipopolysaccharide-induced hepatitis in mice. *Eur J Pharmacol.* 2007 Mar 8;558(1-3):179-84.

Yokoyama M, Yokoyama A, Mori S, Takahashi HK, Yoshino T, Watanabe T, Watanabe T, Ohtsu H, Nishibori M. Inducible histamine protects mice from P. acnes-primed and LPS-induced hepatitis through H2-receptor stimulation. *Gastroenterology.* 2004 Sep;127(3):892-902.

Yoshikawa T, Nakamura T, Yanai K. Histamine N-Methyltransferase in the Brain. *Int J Mol Sci.* 2019 Feb 10;20(3):737. doi: 10.3390/ijms20030737.

Zdravkovic V, Pantovic S, Rosic G, Tomic-Lucic A, Zdravkovic N, Colic M, Obradovic Z, Rosic M. Histamine blood concentration in ischemic heart disease patients. *J Biomed Biotechnol.* 2011;2011:315709.

Zeng Z, Shen L, Li X, Luo T, Wei X, Zhang J, Cao S, Huang X, Fukushima Y, Bin J, Kitakaze M, Xu D, Liao Y. Disruption of histamine H2 receptor slows heart failure progression through reducing myocardial apoptosis and fibrosis. *Clin Sci* (Lond). 2014 Oct;127(7):435-48.

Zhang MZ, Yao B, Wang S, Fan X, Wu G, Yang H, Yin H, Yang S, Harris RC. Intrarenal dopamine deficiency leads to hypertension and decreased longevity in mice. *J Clin Invest.* 2011 Jul;121(7):2845-54. doi: 10.1172/JCI57324.

Zimmermann AS, Burhenne H, Kaever V, Seifert R, Neumann D. Systematic analysis of histamine and N-methylhistamine concentrations in organs from two common laboratory mouse strains: C57Bl/6 and Balb/c. *Inflamm Res.* 2011 Dec;60(12):1153-9.

Zou L, Spanogiannopoulos P, Pieper LM, Chien HC, Cai W, Khuri N, Pottel J, Vora B, Ni Z, Tsakalozou E, Zhang W, Shoichet BK, Giacomini KM, Turnbaugh PJ. Bacterial metabolism rescues the inhibition of intestinal drug absorption by food and drug additives. *Proc Natl Acad Sci U S A.* 2020 Jul 7;117(27):16009-16018. doi: 10.1073/pnas.1920483117.

Chapter 2

IPSCS: A Glimpse into the Future of Clinical Cardiac Tissue Engineering

Alaowei Y. Amanah, Taylor Cook Suh and Jessica M. Gluck,[*] PhD
Textile Engineering, Chemistry and Science,
Wilson College of Textiles, North Carolina State University,
Raleigh, NC, USA

Abstract

Induced pluripotent stem cells (iPSCs) hold the potential to revolutionize cardiac medicine by supplying theoretically limitless quantities of patient-specific cell lines that can provide a more robust and clinically effective diagnosis or treatment. This chapter provides an analytical comparison of iPSCs, mesenchymal stem cells (MSCs), and cardiosphere-derived cells (CDCs) commonly used for clinical cardiac applications. We explore the utilization of iPSCs for cell therapy, including disease modeling, drug screening, and its potential for clinical therapeutic cardiac interventions. The economic, regulatory, legal, and ethical considerations surrounding the use of human iPSCs (hiPSCs) in the clinic are also discussed. Additionally, we delve into the current state of knowledge based on clinical trials and highlight gaps that serve as limitations against clinical applications. Finally, we summarize the outlook and possible futures for iPSCs in clinical cardiac tissue engineering (CTE) applications, which focuses on utilizing cells, growth factors, and scaffolds to construct functional cardiac structures that can

---

[*] Corresponding Author's E-mail: jmgluck@ncsu.edu.

In: Horizons in World Cardiovascular Research. Volume 22
Editor: Eleanor H. Bennington
ISBN: 978-1-68507-568-2

repair or replace damaged tissues, arteries, and the heart. Despite their challenges, such as their metabolic, morphological, and electrophysiological immaturity relative to adult cell lines, iPSCs still provide an exciting and trailblazing opportunity to transform current cardiac clinical standards.

Keywords: induced pluripotent stem cells, clinical cardiac applications, cardiac tissue engineering

Introduction

Cardiac diseases are incredibly complex to treat due to their varying pathophysiological mechanisms making it difficult to develop a standard therapeutic regimen applicable to all subpopulations of patients. As a result, the advent of stem cell therapy as a potential for treating cardiac diseases tailored towards a specific patient population has garnered intense interest over the past two decades. Although it was widely accepted that the heart could not undergo regeneration, research utilizing radiocarbon dating incorporated into DNA to establish the age of cardiomyocytes in humans has shown that cardiomyocytes renew each year at a decreasing rate with age. From age 25 onwards, there is a slow decrease in cardiomyocyte renewal annually from 1% to approximately 0.45% by age 75 (Bergmann et al. 2009, 98–102). Controversial results were published debating the aforementioned sources and generation rates of the cells utilized in the radiocarbon dating study leading to active scientific debate regarding whether cardiomyocyte renewal in adult mammals is in fact plausible (Bergmann and Jovinge 2014, 523–31; Eschenhagen et al. 2017, 680–86). Further studies support the consensus that cardiomyocyte renewal can be achieved either from pre-existing cardiomyocytes that dedifferentiate and duplicate, or via stem cells that can be differentiated to *de novo* cardiomyocytes (Senyo et al. 2013, 433–36; Beltrami et al. 2001, 1750–57; Zebrowski, Becker, and Engel 2016, H1045–54; Park and Yoon 2018, 974). This fuels the current school of thought that it is indeed possible to utilize stem cells to regenerate previously damaged cardiomyocytes (Lázár, Sadek, and Bergmann 2017, 2333–42).

Cardiac renewal typically occurs due to acute stress or chronic pathologies that require the formation of new tissue to promote cardiac repair (Turner et al. 2020, no. 2). According to the world health organization, the leading cause of death globally is myocardial ischemia, which happens to be the most common cardiovascular clinical pathology that stem cell therapy aims to treat (World Health Organization 2020). Myocardial ischemia, colloquially known as coronary artery disease, is reduced blood supply to the heart muscle, leading to a wide array of other diseases such as myocardial infarction (MI), congestive heart failure, and permanent loss or decrease of active cardiomyocytes (Terashvili and Bosnjak 2019, 209–22; Segers and Lee 2008, 937–42). The damaged cardiomyocytes result from a lack of oxygen and blood supply to the myocardium resulting in a range of cardiovascular diseases including MI that require immediate critical care in a clinical setting. Treatment of MI in a controlled clinical setting typically involves the prescription of aspirin to decrease blood clotting and nitro-glycerin or other applicable antihypertensive drugs to ease chest pain and reduce the heart's oxygen demands. In dire cases, physicians recommend an angioplasty surgical intervention to dilate the compressed arteries, coronary bypass surgery to restore blood flow to the heart, or a heart transplant (Lu et al. 2015, 865–67). These existing therapies may lower early mortality rates, prevent further damage to the myocardium, and reduce further risk of redeveloping MI. However, they cannot significantly improve clinical prognosis by replacing permanently damaged cardiomyocytes except for a heart transplant. Still, heart transplants are insufficient for treating MIs because of extensive shortages in available donor organs, long waiting lists, and long-term challenges involving chronic immune rejection of the donated organ (Benjamin et al. 2018, e67–492). Thus, the possibility of utilizing stem cell therapy to fuel cardiac tissue regeneration proves to be an effective therapeutic option because the stem cells can be specifically differentiated into *de novo* cardiomyocytes and used to replace the previously damaged cardiomyocytes (Rao et al., n.d., no. 2). More importantly, the permanently damaged cardiomyocytes caused by the loss of blood and oxygen supply from myocardial ischemia results in the development of fibrous non-contractile scar tissue (J. Li et al. 2020, 8893). Post scar-tissue formation, the affected region experiences impaired function and disruption in action potentials leading to arrhythmias and uncoordinated pumping of the heart. This further initiates a spiral of adverse events that ultimately progress into left ventricular dysfunction or end stage heart failure (J. Li et al. 2020, 8893). By utilizing stem cells to re-muscularize or replace the damaged cardiomyocytes, the efficient and healthy physiological function of the heart can be theoretically restored. Even though there are several different types of stem cells employed in treating MI, this chapter will focus on induced pluripotent stem cells (iPSCs) and provide brief information on the use of mesenchymal stem cells (MSCs) and cardiosphere derived stem cells (CDCs).

Deriving Cardiomyocytes from Induced Pluripotent Stem Cells

Since their discovery, iPSCs have been the center of attention for tissue engineering and regenerative medicine applications due to their theoretical ability to generate limitless quantities of patient-specific cells. In 2006, Takahashi and Yamanaka successfully reprogrammed murine fibroblasts into an embryonic-like state by transducing the transcription factors *Oct3/4, Sox2, c-Myc,* and *Klf4* (Takahashi and Yamanaka 2006, 663–76). The following year, this discovery was translated from mice to humans using the same group of transcription factors (Takahashi et al. 2007, 861–72).

iPSCs are extremely attractive for cardiac tissue engineering and clinical cardiac applications, particularly for their well-established ability to differentiate into cardiomyocytes (CMs). The differentiation of iPSCs to iPSC-CMs has been well understood with optimized protocols since 2012 (Mummery et al. 2012, 344–58; Balafkan et al. 2020, 1–14; Machiraju and Greenway 2019, 33; Talkhabi, Aghdami, and Baharvand 2016, 98–113). This *in vitro* differentiation follows the same sequential stages as embryonic cardiac development. This process is replicated via the use of a specific combination of growth factors to induce cardiogenic mesoderm *in vitro,* causing anteriorly migrated mesoderm cells to switch on a cardiac-specific combination of growth factors that establish the cardiac transcriptional program. Three families of growth factors are thought to control this process: bone morphogenic proteins (BMPs), Wingless-related integration site proteins (WNTs), and fibroblast growth factors (FGFs). Once the cardiac transcriptional program is activated, a highly conserved signaling pathway ensues, involving transcription factors such as the T-box Brachyury, mesoderm posterior 1, and the GATA family of zinc fingers (GATA4/5/6). These transcription factors undergo intricate interactions leading to the differentiation, proliferation, formation, and eventual maturation of CMs from iPSCs. For a thorough understanding of the signaling pathway, see the Mummery et al. 2012 article (Mummery et al. 2012, 344–58).

The maturation of iPSC-CMs is critical for clinical use, as iPSC-CMs are morphologically, electrophysiologically, mechanically, and metabolically immature relative to healthy, functional, adult CMs. Mature CMs exhibit rectangular morphology with highly organized sarcomeres, whereas iPSC-CMs exhibit amorphous or circular morphology with disorganized sarcomeres, and therefore underdeveloped sarcoplasmic reticulum and transverse tubule networks (Huang et al. 2018, 1–4). As a result, excitation-contraction coupling does not occur in iPSC-CMs the way it does *in vivo* due to their immaturity. Overall, iPSC-CMs are so immature that they demonstrate electrical and mechanical properties more similar to embryonic CMs than adult ones (Bruyneel et al. 2018, 55–61). Therefore, it is of critical concern to mature iPSC-CMs before they are clinically used, because their immaturity would prevent them from electrically coupling with mature CMs to propagate action potentials across heart tissue and facilitate beating (Huang et al. 2018, 1–4). Research is currently being conducted to mature iPSC-CMs through a variety of methods including long-term culture, application of electrical stimulation, and mechanical recreation of the heart's pumping physiology (Hirt et al. 2014, 151–61; Lundy et al. 2013, 1991–2002; Liaw and Zimmermann 2016, 156–60).

There are several different methods for initiating *in vitro* differentiation of human iPSCs into iPSC-CMs. Three of the main methods used are embryoid body (EB)-mediated culture, monolayer culture, and inductive co-culture. EB-mediated differentiation was first performed to differentiate human embryonic stem cells (hESCs) to CMs (Vidarsson, Hyllner, and Sartipy 2010, 108–20) and later successfully translated to differentiate CMs from iPSCs (J Zhang 2009, e30–41). In EB-mediated iPSC-CM differentiation, EBs are formed *in vitro* via floating cultivation, and the resultant ball-shaped iPSC structures are transferred to gelatin-coated plates and cultivated (Itskovitz-Eldor et al. 2000, 88–95). This method is inefficient, with a relatively low yield of CM purity less than 1%, and with variable results in downstream differentiation for different iPSC lines (Garbutt, Liu, and Qian 2020, 259–83; Pettinato, Wen, and Zhang 2015, 1595–1609; Parrotta et al. 2020, 4354).

Monolayer culture adds small molecules such as JAK inhibitor I (JAKi) and Rho-kinase inhibitor Y-27632 (ROCKi) into culture media in order to enhance cell adhesion and direct cardiac differentiation of iPSCs (Mummery et al. 2012, 344–58; Batalov and Feinberg 2015, BMI. S20050; Lian et al. 2013, 162–75, 2012, E1848–57; Chen et al. 2012, 237–48). In one adaptation of the monolayer culture differentiation approach, glycogen synthase kinase 3 (GSK3) and WNT inhibitors are used to differentiate iPSCs into CMs via the modulation of WNT and β-catenin signaling in a defined, growth-factor free, and serum-free protocol (Lian et al. 2013, 162–75). This adaptation boasts a yield of up to 85% beating iPSC-CMs (Garbutt, Liu, and Qian 2020, 259–83).

A different adaptation adds the cytokines Activin A, BMP4 and bFGF to the Matrigel coating in order to promote the initial epithelial-mesenchymal transition (EMT) that ultimately leads to mesoderm formation and cardiogenesis (Jianhua Zhang et al. 2010). This adaptation successfully increases the reproducibility of the process and the robustness of the iPSC-CMs generated by monolayer culture differentiation (Mummery et al. 2012, 344–58; Jianhua Zhang et al. 2010), and typically yields greater than 50% beating iPSC-CMs (Garbutt, Liu, and Qian 2020, 259–83).

In the inductive co-culture method, iPSCs are co-cultured with visceral endotherm-like cells to induce their differentiation into CMs. During the co-culture, the small molecule inhibitors of GSK3 and WNT are applied to the cells (Chu et al. 2020, e0230966), similar to what is seen in one of the prominent monolayer differentiation approaches. This protocol is preferred by many because of its low initial cell requirement, rapid progression, and simple execution, as well as the high volume and quality of CMs generated (Le and Chong 2016, 1–4). However, co-culture is often criticized for its low CM yield, which is less than 10% and usually around only 1% (Batalov and Feinberg 2015, BMI. S20050). Many debate which iPSC-CM differentiation method is most effective, but the multiple well-established protocols for production of iPSC-CMs allows for their use in a multitude of cardiac tissue engineering and clinical applications.

Utilization of IPSCs for Cardiovascular Cell Therapies

As mentioned earlier, the use of iPSCs can be advantageous towards counteracting the effects of cardiac pathologies that result from myocardial ischemia, particularly restoring cardiac function to areas of cardiac tissue with excessive scar formation. As a result, clinical indications for iPSC-CMs are promising for cell therapy due to their vast potential for differentiation that can aid in the specific repair of damaged heart valves, vessels, and cardiac muscle tissues (Duelen and Sampaolesi 2017, 30–40). Despite their potential, concerns regarding generating iPSC-CMs that are uniform in cardiac subtype and exhibit mature functional cell characteristics such as efficient calcium handling and myofibril alignment remain present because it limits their ability to serve as true models of adult cardiomyocytes or to replace damaged cardiomyocytes (Duelen and Sampaolesi 2017, 30–40). A lack of efficient calcium handling and myofibril alignment can lead to electrophysiological malfunctions such as spontaneous beating of the iPSC-CMs when not stimulated or inefficient excitation-contraction coupling leading to contractility issues relative to their mature native CM counterparts (J. Li et al. 2020, 8893), namely the development of arrhythmias. If the issues surrounding phenotypic maturity of the iPSC-CMs remain unaddressed, transplantation of the *de novo* generated CMs to scarred areas of the heart to replace damaged cardiomyocytes would be futile because the newly transplanted tissue will be unable to biologically interact with the already existing fully matured adult cells in the heart. Likewise, *in vitro* studies utilizing iPSC-CMs to model diseases affecting cardiac patients may be inadequate if the iPSC-CMs are immature relative to adult CMs (J. Li et al. 2020, 8893). The disease that is modeled cannot be studied past the differentiated stage of the iPSC-CMs. As the disease progresses naturally, information that is retrieved from the study can only be applied to earlier onset stages of the disease creating limitations in therapeutic options for those suffering chronically from the disease.

Regardless of those concerns, iPSC-CMs that were effectively differentiated have successfully provided an avenue for disease modeling and drug screening. For example, *in vitro* models for inherited cardiac diseases, cardiometabolic disorders, and other common cardiomyopathies were successfully modeled by iPSC-CMs(Oikonomopoulos, Kitani, and Wu 2018, 1624–34; Souidi et al. 2020, 102094; Robinton and Daley 2012, 295–305; Bellin et al. 2012, 713–26). With disease modeling, researchers can better investigate and understand the pathognomonic characteristics of cardiovascular diseases that cannot be easily accessed from patients. Some examples of successful disease modeling using hiPSC-CMs include dilated cardiomyopathy and LEOPARD syndrome (Hinson et al. 2015, 982–86; Carvajal-Vergara et al. 2010, 808–12). Furthermore, disease modeling utilizing iPSC-CMs created an opportunity for efficient drug screening by utilizing the *in vitro* models to study gene-drug interactions and drug-induced cardiotoxicity from lifesaving drugs used for other clinical treatments. For example, a well-known drug propranolol, a beta-adrenergic blocking agent, successfully attenuated induced arrhythmia in iPSC-CMs derived and differentiated from patients with Long QT syndromes (Matsa et al. 2011, 952–62). Similarly, research has shown that some highly efficient oncology drugs can lead to cardiac contractile and electrophysiological dysfunction. Thus, the use of *in vitro* hiPSC-CMs can help guide the evaluation of cardiac liabilities and design clinical studies that can illuminate how those drugs negatively affect patients' prognosis (Gintant et al. 2019, e75–92). The potential for clinical therapeutic cardiac interventions using iPSC-CMs in clinical trials still exists. However, issues surrounding genomic instabilities such as single nucleotide variants, copy number variations, and larger chromosomal abnormalities (Martin 2017, 108–17) in iPSC lines and its potential for mutagenesis hindered the application of iPSCs for clinical use (Müller, Lemcke, and David 2018, 2607–55). More importantly, hiPSC-CMs resemble CMs in the embryonic or fetal stage due to lower expressions of maturation-related sarcomeric genes such as MYL2, MYH7, TCAP, and MYOM2, ion transport related genes such as KCNJ2 and RYR2, and the use of glycolysis for energy metabolism as opposed to beta-oxidation of fatty acids (Tang 2020; Di Baldassarre et al. 2018, 48). As mentioned earlier, the immaturity of hiPSC-CMs relative to adult CMs limits their usability as a human cardiomyocyte model posing a challenge to biomedical researchers. Nonetheless, new protocols were developed to address those issues leading to the first wave of clinical trials using iPSCs for treating MI, which will be discussed in the clinical trials section of this chapter. Before we dive into the clinical trials, it is important to provide some important information regarding the regulatory issues hindering biomedical research efforts to utilize iPSCs for treating cardiovascular diseases.

Regulatory Issues Using IPSCs for Cardiac Patients

The current and future uses of iPSCs in the clinic for cardiac-related applications are exciting and hold the potential to revolutionize the field and save many lives by reducing the need for organ and tissue donation, providing *in vitro* diagnostic tools, and opening doors to various treatment options such as regenerative therapies and engineered cardiac tissue. However, there exists economic, regulatory, legal, and ethical considerations that must be addressed before iPSCs can be used in the clinic. Economically, the primary roadblock is the production cost and labor requirement for the development of an iPSC distribution bank. According to a review from Neofytou et al. in 2015, for the effective clinical use of iPSCs, a bank should retain no less than 200-300 vials of cells, with approximately 2 million cells per vial (Neofytou et al. 2015, 2551–57). For numerical context, a group in the U.S. transplanted approximately 750 million cryopreserved human embryonic stem cell-derived cardiomyocytes (hESC-CMs) into macaque monkeys affected with large myocardial infarctions in order to successfully re-muscularize and restore function to the ventricular myocardium (Liu et al. 2018, 597–605). Pre-clinical research suggests that doses up to one billion CMs will be required to achieve the desired therapeutic effects from injection or transplantation (Chong et al. 2014, 273–77; Laflamme and Murry 2005, 845–56). The creation of a bank containing sufficient iPSCs to generate iPSC-CMs in quantities appropriate for tissue engineering applications and clinical applications is very expensive. Many cite the costs at upwards of $800,000 per cell line to develop (Bravery 2015, 1–10). In addition to the procurement of the cell bank itself, Current Good Manufacturing Practices (CGMP) enforced by the U.S. Food and Drug Administration (FDA) require genetic testing and screening for infectious agents including mycoplasma, intracellular bacteria, and viral contaminants (Devito et al. 2014, 1116–24). These processes are costly, and combined with the cost of creating the iPSC bank itself, production quickly enters millions of dollars in price. This creates economic roadblocks for the use of iPSCs in clinical applications.

Despite these economic and logistical challenges, the development of an iPSC cell bank has been shown to be feasible. Japanese researchers are at the cutting edge of this endeavor, aided by the comparatively high level of genetic homogeneity within the Japanese population. In Japan, an iPSC stock project was initiated in 2012 aiming to establish an allogeneic iPSC bank to serve approximately 80% of Japan's population for clinical treatment. The Japanese government invested the equivalent of $275 million USD that year. By 2017, the group had established two cell lines covering 24% of the population, and they aimed to reach 50% coverage by the end of 2020. There was some controversy on the governmental funding of the iPSC stock project in 2012. Notably, at this point, no clinical trials using iPSCs had succeeded yet. Thus, many found this funding premature and unethical (Akabayashi, Nakazawa, and Jecker 2018, 700–702). A breakthrough occurred in 2018, when the world's first commercial iPSC bank opened in Osaka, Japan. The $340 million USD production center generates iPSCs for clinical trials (Daley 2018, 1). The bank deposits clinical-grade iPSC cell lines homozygous for HLA-A, B, and -DR haplotypes which genotypically occur in the Japanese population at a high frequency, thus making the iPSCs produced relevant for clinical use at that high frequency (Ilic 2016). This clearly demonstrates the feasibility of developing iPSC banks to supply cells for clinical applications, though more genetically heterogeneous populations present additional challenges.

Countries with much higher genetic variation, such as the U.S. and the U.K., would require extensive genotyping and exhaustive effort to develop iPSC banks with cell lines capable of serving any meaningful percentage of their populations (Huang et al. 2019, 1–14). The Japanese production center was able to create a stem cell bank serving up to 24% of the population with lines homozygous for HLA-A, -B, and -DR haplotypes because their population has low genetic diversity (Ilic 2016). Conversely, countries with higher genetic diversity would never be able to serve their populations with iPSC lines homozygous for a group of haplotypes so few and specific. Genome-wide profiling performed in the U.K. has revealed that 5-46% of variation in iPSC phenotypes such as differentiation capacity and cellular morphology is due to differences between individuals. They therefore concluded that genetic variation drives molecular heterogeneity within human iPSC lines (Kilpinen et al. 2017, 370–75). This heterogeneity must be addressed in order for iPSC banks to be feasible sources for clinical applications within countries whose populations have high genetic diversity.

Regulatory hurdles also pose challenges to the clinical implementation of iPSCs. A primary concern is that autologously harvested iPSC-CMs have large variability between different cell lines (Bravery 2015, 1–10). This variability arises due to differences in donor cell sources, collection methods, and reprogramming techniques. Establishment of standard production protocols is therefore difficult, and such processes are required to satisfy regulatory agencies such as the FDA. This variability also accounts for safety concerns that may delay clinical cardiac-related use of iPSCs for time-sensitive treatments, such as acute myocardial infarction. Many argue that an HLA-matched allogeneic cell bank would address these issues, as it would allow for standardization of production and tissue source (Prescott 2011, 2323–28).

There are also legal considerations for the use of iPSCs in the clinic. Such legal considerations include the manufacturing conditions required to produce clinical-grade iPSCs, the privacy concerns surrounding genetic material as confidential personal information, the feasibility of acquiring fully informed consent from patients, the legality of genetically manipulating autologously harvested iPSCs, and concerns regarding intellectual property and patents (Moradi et al. 2019, 1–13). Although iPSCs are generally considered less ethically controversial than embryonic stem cells, they are still the center of much ethical debate, especially in the context of clinical use. Many of the aforementioned legal considerations, especially informed consent, personal ownership over one's genetic material, and privacy concerns, also introduce ethical questions.

A historical example where these ethical questions were not addressed is the acquisition and use of HeLa cells. The HeLa cell line was nonconsensually taken from Henrietta Lacks, a 30-year-old African American woman who presented with cervical cancer at Johns Hopkins University in 1951, and died due to the cancer that same year. Her cancer cells, now referred to as HeLa cells, were discovered to be capable of indefinite survival and proliferation in culture. These cells are used ubiquitously to this day in cancer research and have made many breakthroughs possible. However, the fact remains that informed consent was not acquired from Henrietta Lacks regarding the use of cells from her tissue for research, her rights and ownership over her own genetic material, and the privacy concerns surrounding the harvesting of her cells (Beskow 2016, 395–417; Times 2013, 1073). This serves as an important example of the need to seriously address these considerations when moving forward with iPSC research, as iPSCs are also taken from patients.

Clinical Trials Using IPSCs

Despite the regulatory issues surrounding the use of iPSCs for cardiac patients, clinical trials currently utilizing hiPSCs for cardiac indications were recently approved. However, only a few trials have been approved due to the aforementioned risks involved with using hiPSCs. One such study in phase 1 involves evaluating the efficacy and safety of a hiPSC-CM patch in combination with an immunosuppressant for patients with severe myocardial ischemia (clinicaltrials.gov ID NCT04696328). The research team hopes that the surgical implantation of the 100 million reprogrammed hiPSC-CMs will help regenerate the damaged heart tissue by releasing growth factors; however, results from the study have yet to be published as the estimated completion study is set for 2023 (Cyranoski 2018, 619). Another currently approved clinical trial in China is the Treating Heart Failure with hPSC-CMs (HEAL-CHF) that was recruiting 5 participants for epicardial injection with allogeneic hPSC-CMS during a coronary artery bypass graft surgery to assess the safety and efficacy of the transplantation after 3, 6, and 12 months. Due to the impacts of the COVID-19 pandemic, updates to this study have not been published despite an estimated completion date in 2020 (clinicaltrials.gov ID NCT03763136). Another clinical trial in Germany studying the safety and efficacy of IPSC-derived Engineered Human Myocardium (EHM) as Biological Ventricular Assist Tissue in Terminal Heart Failure (BioVAT-HF) is currently underway and recruiting approximately 53 patients to test the hypothesis that the EHM BioVAT will lead to re-muscularization of the failing heart and improved myocardial function. The target population for this clinical trial is patients suffering from advanced heart failure with a reduced ejection fraction of less than 35% with no prospect for a heart transplant. Similar to the other studies above, no results have been posted as the estimated completion date for this study is in 2024 (clinicaltrials.gov ID NCT04396899). At this time, there are no further approved clinical trials utilizing hIPSC-CMs implantation for treating debilitating cardiac diseases.

Mesenchymal Stem Cells (MSCs)

iPSCs are not the only type of cell explored and used for cardiac clinical applications. In fact, the field is encouraged to explore iPSCs in part because of the history of use of MSC for cardiac-related applications. MSCs have been used successfully in cell therapies for a wide variety of organs and tissues in clinical trials. MSCs were first explored for cellular and regenerative therapies for skeletal tissue repairs. Clinical trials were conducted on allogeneic bone marrow-derived MSCs transplants for the treatment of osteogenesis imperfecta, Hurler syndrome, and metachromatic leukodystrophy (Lazarus et al. 1995, 557–64; Koç et al. 2000, 307; Horwitz et al. 2001, 1227–31, 2002, 8932–37). Early focus on MSCs for clinical use almost exclusively explored skeletal applications due to the assumption that because MSCs functioned as stromal cells, they would be most effective in for therapies related to connective and hematopoietic tissue (Parekkadan and Milwid 2010, 87–117; Musiał-Wysocka, Kot, and Majka 2019, 801–12). Clinical trials later expanded to explore the use of MSCs for the treatment of steroid-resistant graft vs. host disease, Chrohn's disease, type I diabetes mellitus, myocardial infarction, and chronic obstructive pulmonary disease (Parekkadan and Milwid 2010, 87–117). Interestingly, there is also research that derives MSCs from iPSCs, and uses them to treat steroid-resistant graft vs. host disease, induce immune tolerance following tracheal implants, repair acute kidney injury, recover endometrial tissue, and more (Bloor et al. 2020, 1720–25; Khan et al. 2019, 1–15; Huang, Wang, and Xu 2020, 204–9; Ji et al. 2020, 268–84).

Stem cells are defined by their capacity to self-renew via division and to differentiate into multi-lineage cells. Stem cells are categorized as pluripotent (including iPSC) or adult stem cells, which exhibit lower potency (i.e., differentiation potential) than pluripotent stem cells, meaning they are only capable of differentiating into a limited number of specific cell types (multipotent) (Bacakova et al. 2018, 1111–26). Mesenchymal stem cells (MSCs) are a type of adult stem cells. In addition to iPSCs, these MSCs are also of interest for clinical cardiac applications. MSCs demonstrate multipotency, capable of differentiating into the mesodermal lineages of osteocytes, adipocytes, and chondrocytes; the ectodermal lineage of neurocytes; and the endodermal lineage of hepatocytes (Ullah, Subbarao, and Rho 2015a, no. 2). Such MSCs are attractive due to their multipotency, immunomodulation, and secretion of anti-inflammatory molecules. These characteristics endow them with the ability to regulate microenvironments, which is crucial in achieving microenvironmental biomimicry (Ullah, Subbarao, and Rho 2015a, no. 2). This biomimicry is critical for cardiac applications because the microenvironment of the cells is intended to recapitulate aspects of the *in vivo* environment. By doing so, this allows the production of *in vitro* culture systems that promote the physiological maturation of differentiated stem cells closely resembling and functioning similarly to the cells found in the human body (Smith et al. 2017, 77–94). Though first discovered when acquired from bone marrow tissue (Pittenger et al. 1999a, 143–47), MSCs have since successfully been isolated from almost all tissues in the human body (Crisan et al. 2008, 301–13). Additionally, it has been shown that MSCs can be derived from pluripotent stem cells, including iPSCs and ESCs (Zhang et al. 2015, 1–17; Miao et al. 2014, 1644–54). MSCs are defined by three criteria: positive expression of CD73, D90, and CD105 with negative expression of CD14, CD34, CD45, and HLA-DR; adherence to plastic under standard culture conditions; and retention of *in vitro* multi-lineage multipotency including adipogenic, chondrogenic, and osteogenic (Ullah, Subbarao, and Rho 2015b, no. 2; Kobayashi and Suzuki 2018, 2222–32; Pittenger et al. 1999b, 143–47).

Comparing iPSCs to MSCs reveals many similarities and differences. MSCs and iPSCs are both amenable to autologous transplantation, which is greatly preferred in the clinic because it avoids the immune responses associated with rejection (Sachs et al. 2012, 505–15). iPSCs and MSCs are also similar in that both boast a diverse range of sources. MSCs and iPSCs differ in their morphology, phenotype, plasticity, differentiation potential, and tumorigenesis. MSCs exhibit a fibroblast-like morphology (Webster et al. 2012, 265–72), whereas iPSCs exhibit an embryonic stem cell-like (Takahashi and Yamanaka 2006, 663–76). Phenotypically, iPSCs and MSCs exhibit different genetic markers and transcription factors, as shown in Table 1 below (Zomer et al. 2015, 125; Xu et al. 2019, 754–65; Ledesma-Martínez, Mendoza-Núñez, and Santiago-Osorio 2016, vol. 2016). iPSCs are pluripotent, whereas MSCs are multipotent. As a result, iPSCs exhibit the potential to differentiate into endodermal, mesodermal, and ectodermal tissues, but MSCs are only capable of differentiating into mesodermal tissues, as well as neurocytes from the ectoderm and hepatocytes from the endoderm. Finally, iPSCs exhibit tumorigenesis, and MSCs do not (Insausti et al. 2014, 53).

Though MSCs offer many distinct advantages for clinical cardiac applications, they are not without challenges. Most problematic is their loss of potency during *in vitro* sub-culturing at higher passages, which prevents them from expanding into the quantities necessary for clinical use. Large quantities of MSCs are needed to meet the engraftment, structural organization, and cellular differentiation requirements necessary to repair or replace damaged cardiac tissue (Pittenger et al. 2019, 1–15). It is important to note that iPSCs displaying a greater differentiation potential, as highlighted in table 2, may contribute to differences in ease of deriving CMs from iPSCs when compared to MSCs. Regardless, to address MSCs loss of potency, research suggests that doses of up to one billion CMs are needed to successfully achieve therapeutic results in the clinic from injection or transplantation of cells to treat cardiac issues (Chong et al. 2014, 273–77; Laflamme and Murry 2005, 845–56). MSCs' *in vitro* loss of potency occurs primarily due to decreased telomerase activity (Kassem 2004, 369–74). Additionally, long-term *in vitro* culture of MSCs has been shown to degrade their multipotency via alterations in their epigenetic profiles, specifically their CpG methylation patterns, and increase their susceptibility to malignant transformation (Røsland et al. 2009, 5331–39; de Almeida et al. 2016, 168–75). For example, MSCs derived from bone marrow exhibit senescence during long-term culture, resulting in decreased differentiation potential, shortened telomere length, and altered morphology (Bonab et al. 2006, 1–7).

Table 1. Comparison of iPSCs and MSCs

Characteristics	**Cell Type**	
	iPSCs	MSCs
Morphology	Embryonic stem cell-like	Fibroblast-like
Markers	OCT4+, NANOG+, SOX2+, SSEA1+, SSEA3+, SSEA4+, TRA1-60+, TRA1-81+, ALP+	CD29+, CD44+, CD73+, CD90+, CD105+, CD166+, CD14−, CD31−, CD45−, CD34
Potency	Pluripotent	Multipotent
Differentiation Potential	Endodermal, mesodermal, ectodermal	Mesodermal, neurocytes from ectoderm, hepatocytes from endoderm
Tumorigenesis	Exhibited	Not exhibited

Clinical Trials Using MSCs

Specific to cardiac clinical applications, MSCs are relevant because there is much research done on their capacity to differentiate into cardiomyocytes and their injection into the heart to treat myocardial infarction and other pathologies. In 2013, a research team reported successful differentiation of perinatally-derived MSCs into CM-like cells (Nartprayut et al. 2013, 1465–69). Studies have shown that bone-marrow derived MSCs are capable of trans-differentiating into CMs *in vitro* via treatment with co-culture with rodent CMs or treatment with 5-azacytidine (Makino et al. 1999, 697–705; Fukuda 2001, 187–93; Yoon et al. 2005, 715–21; Shi et al. 2016, vol. 2016; Xu et al. 2004, 623–31). Bone marrow-derived MSC-CMs are commonly used in animal research focused on myocardial repair via cell transplantation. For example, autologous trans-differentiated MSC-CMs have been delivered via fibrin patches to pigs for post-infarction left ventricular remodeling and shown to further differentiate into cells with CM-like characteristics as well as significantly increase neovascularization *in vivo* (Liu et al. 2004, H501–11). The successes of such studies indicate promise for MSC-CMs in clinical cardiac applications for the treatment of myocardial infarction and heart failure.

In addition to their differentiation into MSC-CMs for cardiac clinical applications, MSCs themselves have shown promise in treating myocardial infarction when injected. Therapeutic injections of MSCs have shown the capability to reverse myocardial injury and improve cardiac function. Left ventricular function is considered the gold standard surrogate endpoint to assess efficacy of heart failure treatments, and left ventricular remodeling is an independent predictor of cardiovascular mortality (Jin et al. 2010, 249–53). Clinical trials have demonstrated that MSCs when injected are safe and successful in increasing left ventricular function, thus making MSC injections an attractive therapy for myocardial infarction (Banerjee, Bolli, and Hare 2018, 266–87). MSCs have also been shown to ameliorate cardiovascular diseases due to their immunoregulatory abilities, antifibrotic effects, and neovascularization features. Their mode of therapeutic function towards these cardiovascular diseases is primarily paracrine-based (Y. Guo et al. 2020, 1–10). The paracrine effect of MSCs for cardiovascular tissue repair requires further investigation because it brings into question whether the number of cells injected into the injured site and their engraftment within that site plays a vital role in therapeutic efficacy. Low cardiac engraftment rates from MSC studies coupled with the paracrine effect of MSCs show that the cells in-fact may not be solely responsible for the observed improved cardiovascular function (Hare et al. 2009a, 2277–86; Mirotsou et al. 2011, 280–89). Post intracoronary injection of MSCs, the cells extravasate and engraft into the injured site. During that process, some of the cells may be lost after stimulating repair via paracrine signaling. As a result, the future of cell-based therapies may involve treatment with cell-free suspensions of paracrine molecules produced by stem cells to stimulate immune-related repair of cardiovascular diseases, and to determine the impact of the presence of the cells in definitively treating the injured site (Banerjee, Bolli, and Hare 2018, 266–87).

Research has shown that MSCs regulate inflammatory response via immunomodulatory processes that suppress white blood cells and trigger anti-inflammatory pathways in both innate and adaptive immunities (Chiossone et al. 2016, 1909–21; Najar et al. 2016, 160–71). MSCs have been shown to bolster these immune responses via paracrine mechanisms which reduce apoptosis of myocardial cells, levels of inflammatory cytokines and monocyte chemotactic protein-1 (MCP-1), and MCP-1-mediated damage to cardiac cells (J. Guo et al. 2007, 97–104; Ohnishi et al. 2007, 88–97). Additionally, bone marrow-derived MSCs have demonstrated the ability to inhibit secretion of antigen-specific immunoglobulins M and G1, thereby suppressing B-cell terminal differentiation (Asari et al. 2009, 604–15). These paracrine effects which enhance innate and adaptive immune responses make MSCs attractive for clinical implementation in the treatment of cardiac causes.

The first clinical trials using MSCs to treat myocardial infarction delivered intracoronary autologous MSCs during percutaneous coronary intervention and demonstrated that the MSCs significantly increased left ventricular function, increased exercise capacity, and improved in a heart failure class, with no serious adverse effects (Chen et al. 2004, 92–95). This trial occurred in 2014 by Chen et al. in China. Other clinical trials that followed similarly demonstrated the safety and efficacy of intracoronary delivery of MSCs to improve left ventricular function following myocardial infarction (Katritsis et al. 2007, 167–71; Williams et al. 2011a, 792–96; MOHY et al. 2007). In 2009, a randomized, double-blind, placebo-controlled, dose-escalation clinical trial intravenously delivered allogeneic MSCs to 53 patients after acute myocardial infarction and found no adverse effects compared to the placebo group. Furthermore, it was found that the MSC-treated patients experienced reduction in ventricular tachycardia episodes, improvement in pulmonary function, and most importantly, significantly improved left ventricular ejection fraction, corresponding to improved left ventricular function (Hare et al. 2009b, 2277–86). This trial heralded an era of equal focus on allogeneic and autologous MSCs for clinical cardiac applications, whereas previously the field was dominated by autologous MSCs (White et al. 2016, 55–87). In 2013, a group compared allogeneic vs. autologous bone marrow-derived MSCs in a randomized dose-escalation trial which transendocardially injected 20, 100, or 200 million allogeneic or autologous MSCs into patients with ischemic cardiomyopathy. The trial revealed that both allogeneic and autologous bone marrow-derived MSCs were safe and reduced scar sizes by 33.21%, that allogeneic MSCs reduced left ventricular end-diastolic volumes, that allogeneic MSCs did not stimulate significant donor-specific alloimmune reactions, and that the lowest concentration of injected MSCs resulted in the greatest increase in left ventricular function (Hare et al. 2012, 2369–79).

Clinical trials using MSCs for cardiac applications have also demonstrated that MSCs functionally restitute and thus improve function of the left ventricle when injected together with Coronary Artery Bypass Grafting (Karantalis et al. 2014, 1302–10), improve regional contractility and reduce scar size when injected into patients with cardiomyopathy (Williams et al. 2011b, 792–96), and improve left ventricular ejection fraction when injected into patients using a Left Ventricular Mechanical Support Device, even when the device was turned off (Anastasiadis et al. 2012, e51–53).

It is widely thought that MSCs are so effective in left ventricular remodeling and improving left ventricular and cardiovascular function because they are believed to derive from the mesoderm, from which the cells that form the myocardium are also derived (White et al. 2016, 55–87). MSCs are strong mediators of cardiac repair, and thus highly explored for both preclinical research and clinical trials in the treatment of cardiac diseases, particularly, as discussed, myocardial infarction.

According to clinicaltrials.gov as of June 2021, there are currently 135 registered clinical trials globally using MSCs for cardiac-related research. In Korea, researchers assessed the safety and efficacy of intracoronary injections of MSCs into 80 participants aged 18-70 to treat acute myocardial infarction (Lee et al. 2014, 23). A similar clinical trial is being conducted in Spain, but the MSCs were delivered instead using a decellularized matrix intended to transport the cells directly to the myocardial infarction (clinicaltrials.gov ID NCT03798353). In Colombia, a clinical trial seeks to evaluate the safety of intramyocardial injection of Wharton's jelly-derived MSCs to increase cardiac function and myocardial viability, as well as reduce ventricular arrhythmias within infarcted heart tissue (clinicaltrials.gov ID NCT04011059). In the U.S., a clinical trial transendocardially injected 20 million, 100 million, or 200 million autologous or allogeneic MSCs during cardiac catheterization to repair and regenerate damaged myocardia (clinicaltrials.gov ID NCT01087996). Other clinical trials in the U.S. intravenously infuse allogeneic MSCs to treat heart failure secondary to the complications from the chemotherapy drug Anthracyclines (clinicaltrials.gov ID NCT02408432), assess the effect of MSC injection on neomyogenesis in dilated cardiomyopathy (clinicaltrials.gov ID NCT01392625), and transendocardially inject autologous MSCs and bone marrow cells (BMCs) to treat ischemic heart failure (clinicaltrials.gov ID NCT00768066).

Table 2. Clinical trials involving the use of MSCs
to treat cardiac diseases

clinicaltrials.gov ID	Cells	Aim
NCT01392105	MSCs via intracoronary injection	Assess safety and efficacy for treatment of myocardial infarction
NCT03798353	MSCs delivered via decellularized matrix	Transport MSCs to site of infarction to treat
NCT04011059	Wharton's jelly-derived MSCs via injection	Assess safety if MSC injection to increase cardiac function and myocardial viability
NCT01087996	MSCs delivered during cardiac catheterization	Repair and regenerate damaged myocardium
NCT02408432	MSCs via intravenous infusion	Treat heart failure occurring secondary to complications due to the chemotherapy drug Anthracyclines
NCT01392625	MSCs via injection	Assess effect on neomyogenesis in dilated cardiomyopathy
NCT00768066	Bone marrow-derived MSCs via transendocardial injection	Treat ischemic heart failure

Clearly, most clinical trials focus on the injection of MSCs to treat myocardial infarction and heart failure. This is because MSCs when injected into the myocardium have been shown to exhibit cardiac reparative and regenerative properties, potential for CM differentiation (Mokino and Fududa 1999, 103), engraftment (Pittenger et al. 1999, 143–47), tissue elasticity restoration (Berry et al. 2006, H2196–2203), release of cytokines and growth factors that facilitate endogenous repair mechanism, reduce inducible ventricular tachycardias, increase action potential duration, remodel gap junctions, and ameliorate interstitial fibrosis (Wang et al. 2011, 314–20). However, the mechanism behind many of these processes is not fully understood, and there have been clinical trials showing the failure of bone marrow cells to engraft into infarcted tissue and reduce infarction sizes, leading to many questioning rather bone marrow-derived MSCs will be capable of doing so *in vivo* (Amado et al. 2005, 11474–79).

Cardiosphere-Derived Cells (CDCs)

Another major clinical cell type for cardiac applications is cardiosphere-derived cells (CDCs). CDCs are promising for these applications because they, like iPSCs, offer patient specificity. They offer a distinct advantage over iPSCs because they are more readily available. CDCs can be harvested from cardiac muscle biopsies during surgery (Emani and Del Nido 2018). Thus, unlike iPSCs, they do not require cell line derivation and development of cell banks, circumventing many of the challenges described earlier in the Regulatory Issues section. Interestingly, the success of CDCs in clinical cardiac therapeutics due to their pluripotency suggests that iPSCs will similarly be successful due to their pluripotency (Abou-Saleh et al. 2018, 1–31; Constantinou et al. 2020, 1–18; T.-S. Li et al. 2012a, 942–53).

Cardiospheres are spherical aggregates of cells grown from heart biopsies which self-assemble into clusters in suspension culture (Davis, Smith, and Marbán 2010, 903). They comprise a core of primitive proliferating cells surrounded by a layer of mesenchymal cells and differentiating cells expressing cardiac-specific proteins. CDCs inherently contain all three major cell types present in the human heart - CMs, endothelial cells, and smooth cells (Barile et al. 2013, vol. 2013). CDCs are extremely attractive for cardiac tissue engineering and clinical applications. Research has shown that CDCs, when delivered to infarcted hearts, reduce scarring, decrease infarct size, increase viable myocardium, and improve cardiac function in animal studies (T. Li et al. 2010, 2088–98; Johnston et al. 2009, 1075–83; Messina et al. 2004, 911–21; Leppo et al. 2007). CDCs exhibit higher myogenic differentiation rates than both MSCs and iPSCs, as well as ESCs (Barile et al. 2013, vol. 2013; Menasché 2015, 20140373; T.-S. Li et al. 2012b, 942–53). Interestingly, research has shown that microscale generation of cardiospheres promotes robust enrichment of iPSC-CMs. CMs from cardiospheres were enriched up to approximately 100%. CMs within the cardiospheres exhibited enhanced sarcomeric structure and function compared to those from parallel monolayer culture. This enrichment is hypothesized to be mediated via selective cell survival and homophilic association (Nguyen et al. 2014, 260–68). Despite their many advantages, CDCs are far from without challenges of their own. Most notably, though transplanted CDCs do consistently differentiate into cardiac cells, the long-term persistence of the transplanted CDCs is relatively low and partially depends on paracrine effects for the aforementioned results (Chimenti et al. 2010, 971–80).

Clinical Trials Using CDCs

The first clinical use of CDCs occurred in the CArdiosphere-Derived aUtologous stem cElls to reverse ventricUlar dySfunction (CADUCEUS) trial in the U.S., from which the first paper was published in 2012 (Makkar et al. 2012, 895–904) and the summation of the one-year trial was published in 2014 (Malliaras et al. 2014, 110–22). The CADUCEUS trial tested the safety and efficacy of CDCs by infusing CDCs autologously grown from endomyocardial biopsies into patients 2-4 weeks post-myocardial infarction. This treatment was compared to routine care controls using randomly allocated patients (Makkar et al. 2012, 895–904). The trial was conducted over one year, at the end of which it was concluded that there was no significant difference in safety endpoints (death, ventricular fibrillation, additional myocardial infarction, new cardiac tumor formation, and major adverse cardiac event) between CDC and control groups. Furthermore, MRIs revealed that the CDC-treated group exhibited significant reduction in scar mass at 6- and 12-months post-treatment, whereas the control group did not (Malliaras et al. 2014, 110–22). The CADUCEUS trial was groundbreaking, showing that over the course of 1-year post-treatment, autologous CDC infusion presented no adverse effects outside the realm of those experienced from the control, and significantly reduced scar mass in comparison.

According to clinicaltrials.gov as of June 2021, there are 17 clinical trials globally registered using CDCs currently. They aim to treat myocardial infarction, pulmonary arterial hypertension, Duchenne muscular dystrophy, dilated cardiomyopathy, ischemic cardiomyopathy, non-ischemic cardiomyopathy, coronary artery disease, COVID-19, and heart failure (clinicaltrials.gov).

Outlook and Possible Future for iPSCs in Cardiac Tissue Engineering Applications

Clinical trials involving iPSCs, MSCs, and CDCs to treat cardiac diseases were approved, showing a shift in paradigm for how cardiac care can be delivered. More importantly, the potential for iPSCs to transform the delivery of cardiac medicine cannot be overlooked, given the recent advances to improve the application of such cells in a clinical setting. One such advancement is applying iPSCs in cardiac tissue engineering (CTE) (Smith et al. 2017, 77–94). CTE involves constructing functional cardiac tissues that can repair or replace damaged portions of the heart through a successful combination of cardiac cells, growth factors, and scaffolds. As mentioned earlier, the complexity involved in developing a standard therapeutic regimen for cardiac diseases applicable to all subpopulations of patients can be addressed by using iPSCs for CTE because it circumvents the issue of immunogenicity given that the cells used can be autologously derived. In other words, they are obtained from the same individual receiving the CTE treatment. As a result, it provides the perfect avenue for personalized therapeutic models and patient-specific treatment. Since its discovery, various research teams have been continuously developing protocols to optimize the development of iPSC-based CTE either by using different biomaterials for scaffold development or introducing iPSCs to 3D-engineered cardiac tissue models amongst other approaches (Smith et al. 2017, 77–94; Mazzola and Di Pasquale 2020, vol. 8). The advantages of using CTE to treat cardiac diseases rely on the high biocompatibility and mimicry of the native myocardium *in vivo*.

Earlier, we discussed how iPSCs were successfully used for disease modeling and drug screening in traditional cell line assays for specific cardiac diseases *in vitro*. However, other multisystem organ diseases can cause debilitating cardiac defects such as connective tissue disorders. For example, scleroderma has multiple cardiac manifestations such as MI, fibrosis of the heart chambers leading to left ventricular diastolic dysfunction, and conduction system diseases such as arrhythmias even though it is not a cardiac-specific disease (Mukherjee et al., n.d.; Champion 2008, 181–90; Butt et al. 2019, e013405). Looking ahead, integrating iPSC-based CTE systems with other cell types that can negatively affect the physiological function of the heart can enable more accurate comparisons with the *in vivo* conditions. A scleroderma iPSC-based model of the myocardium is an example of a potential future direction CTE can take to provide more excellent in-depth analysis of how connective tissue disorders can contribute to cardiac defects. Given the prevalence of heart diseases globally, this can lead to more accurate analysis and precise modeling of cell-cell and cell-matrix interactions mirroring the *in-vivo* interactions of how other diseases affect the physiological function of the heart (Smith et al. 2017, 77–94).

Despite the excitement surrounding iPSC-based CTE systems, limitations do exist. The limitations of the regenerative potential of iPSC-CMs within CTE systems are due to their metabolic, morphological, and electrophysiological immaturity relative to adult cell lines (Huang et al. 2018, 1–4). To address this limitation, there is an increase in bioengineering strategies targeted towards improving the development of CTE through manipulation of the ECM alignment and topography, enhancing the scaffold's adherence to the cells, electrochemical stimulation to improve differentiation and maturation of cultured CMs, and small molecule doping (Smith et al. 2017, 77–94). Chronic electrical stimulation of iPSC-based CTE systems was shown to have positive effects on cardiomyocyte density, contractile force production, and sarcomere development (Hirt et al. 2014, 151–61). To address the issues surrounding cardiac phenotype, the use of thyroid hormone T3 on iPSC-CMs upregulated cardiac contractile markers correlating with improved calcium handling and increased force production (Yang et al. 2014, 296–304). The biomedical engineering and research community are consistently developing more solutions to improve how the cells interact with each other and the scaffolds in CTE to transform our understanding of cardiac diseases today.

By constructing more sophisticated and thorough methods that account for their differences to adult cell lines, iPSCs may be approved to the extent of MSCs, given their similarities. In a positive light, the clinical trials using iPSCs mentioned earlier in this chapter are a testament to the potential iPSC-based CTE applications have on treating cardiac diseases. As the results of those trials become available and improved CTE systems are developed, we can expect to see the unveiling of the bright future iPSCs hold in treating cardiac diseases currently responsible for ending millions of lives.

Conclusion

The widespread acceptance of iPSCs in biomedical research is beneficial towards increasing our understanding of cardiac disease progression, drug development, and the clinical treatment of cardiac diseases. The current utilization of iPSCs for patient specific disease modeling based on their genetic backgrounds, drug screening for cardiotoxicity, and in combination with biomaterials for CTE in clinical trials are the tip of the iceberg regarding how iPSCs can transform cardiac medicine. There is much left to explore such as improving cardiac modeling of iPSCs by developing standardized protocols that addresses the issue of maturation relative to adult CMs, as well as analysis of the results of the clinical trials to assess areas for further improvement.

References

Abou-Saleh, Haissam, Fouad A. Zouein, Ahmed El-Yazbi, Despina Sanoudou, Christophe Raynaud, Christopher Rao, Gianfranco Pintus, Hassan Dehaini, and Ali H. Eid. 2018. "The March of Pluripotent Stem Cells in Cardiovascular Regenerative Medicine." *Stem Cell Research & Therapy* 9 (1): 1-31.

Akabayashi, Akira, Eisuke Nakazawa, and Nancy S. Jecker. 2018. "Endangerment of the iPSC Stock Project in Japan: On the Ethics of Public Funding Policies." *Journal of Medical Ethics* 44 (10): 700-702.

Amado, Luciano C., Anastasios P. Saliaris, Karl H. Schuleri, Marcus St, John, Jin-Sheng Xie, Stephen Cattaneo, et al. 2005. "Cardiac Repair with Intramyocardial Injection of Allogeneic Mesenchymal Stem Cells after Myocardial Infarction." *Proceedings of the National Academy of Sciences - PNAS* 102 (32): 11474-11479. doi:10.1073/pnas.0504388102. https://www.jstor.org/stable/3376291.

Anastasiadis, Kyriakos, Polychronis Antonitsis, Argirios Doumas, Georgios Koliakos, Helena Argiriadou, Christina Vaitsopoulou, Paschalis Tossios, Christos Papakonstantinou, and Stephen Westaby. 2012. "Stem Cells Transplantation Combined with Long-Term Mechanical Circulatory Support Enhances Myocardial Viability in End-Stage Ischemic Cardiomyopathy." *International Journal of Cardiology* 155 (3): e51-e53.

Asari, Sadaki, Shin Itakura, Kevin Ferreri, Chih-Pin Liu, Yoshikazu Kuroda, Fouad Kandeel, and Yoko Mullen. 2009. "Mesenchymal Stem Cells Suppress B-Cell Terminal Differentiation." *Experimental Hematology* 37 (5): 604-615.

Bacakova, Lucie, Jana Zarubova, Martina Travnickova, Jana Musilkova, Julia Pajorova, Petr Slepicka, Nikola Slepickova Kasalkova, Vaclav Svorcik, Zdenka Kolska, and Hooman Motarjemi. 2018. "Stem Cells: Their Source, Potency and use in Regenerative Therapies with Focus on Adipose-Derived Stem Cells–a Review." *Biotechnology Advances* 36 (4): 1111-1126.

Balafkan, Novin, Sepideh Mostafavi, Manja Schubert, Richard Siller, Kristina Xiao Liang, Gareth Sullivan, and Laurence A. Bindoff. 2020. "A Method for

Differentiating Human Induced Pluripotent Stem Cells Toward Functional Cardiomyocytes in 96-Well Microplates." *Scientific Reports* 10 (1): 1-14.

Banerjee, Monisha N., Roberto Bolli, and Joshua M. Hare. 2018. "Clinical Studies of Cell Therapy in Cardiovascular Medicine: Recent Developments and Future Directions." *Circulation Research* 123 (2): 266-287.

Barile, Lucio, Mihaela Gherghiceanu, Laurenţiu M. Popescu, Tiziano Moccetti, and Giuseppe Vassalli. 2013. "Human Cardiospheres as a Source of Multipotent Stem and Progenitor Cells." *Stem Cells International* 2013.

Batalov, Ivan and Adam W. Feinberg. 2015. "Differentiation of Cardiomyocytes from Human Pluripotent Stem Cells using Monolayer Culture: Supplementary Issue: Stem Cell Biology." *Biomarker Insights* 10: BMI. S20050.

Bellin, Milena, Maria C. Marchetto, Fred H. Gage, and Christine L. Mummery. 2012. "Induced Pluripotent Stem Cells: The New Patient?" *Nature Reviews Molecular Cell Biology* 13 (11): 713-726.

Beltrami, Antonio P., Konrad Urbanek, Jan Kajstura, Shao-Min Yan, Nicoletta Finato, Rossana Bussani, Bernardo Nadal-Ginard, Furio Silvestri, Annarosa Leri, and C. Alberto Beltrami. 2001. "Evidence that Human Cardiac Myocytes Divide After Myocardial Infarction." *New England Journal of Medicine* 344 (23): 1750-1757.

Benjamin, Emelia J., Salim S. Virani, Clifton W. Callaway, Alanna M. Chamberlain, Alexander R. Chang, Susan Cheng, Stephanie E. Chiuve, Mary Cushman, Francesca N. Delling, and Rajat Deo. 2018. "Heart Disease and Stroke statistics—2018 Update: A Report from the American Heart Association." *Circulation* 137 (12): e67-e492.

Bergmann, Olaf, Ratan D. Bhardwaj, Samuel Bernard, Sofia Zdunek, Fanie Barnabé-Heider, Stuart Walsh, Joel Zupicich, Kanar Alkass, Bruce A. Buchholz, and Henrik Druid. 2009. "Evidence for Cardiomyocyte Renewal in Humans." *Science* 324 (5923): 98-102.

Bergmann, Olaf and Stefan Jovinge. 2014. "Cardiac Regeneration in Vivo: Mending the Heart from within?" *Stem Cell Research* 13 (3): 523-531.

Berry, Mark F., Adam J. Engler, Y. Joseph Woo, Timothy J. Pirolli, Lawrence T. Bish, Vasant Jayasankar, Kevin J. Morine, Timothy J. Gardner, Dennis E. Discher, and H. Lee Sweeney. 2006. "Mesenchymal Stem Cell Injection After Myocardial Infarction Improves Myocardial Compliance." *American Journal of Physiology-Heart and Circulatory Physiology* 290 (6): H2196-H2203.

Beskow, Laura M. 2016. "Lessons from HeLa Cells: The Ethics and Policy of Biospecimens." *Annual Review of Genomics and Human Genetics* 17: 395-417.

Bloor, Adrian JC, Amit Patel, James E. Griffin, Maria H. Gilleece, Rohini Radia, David T. Yeung, Diana Drier, Laurie S. Larson, Gene I. Uenishi, and Derek

Hei. 2020. "Production, Safety and Efficacy of iPSC-Derived Mesenchymal Stromal Cells in Acute Steroid-Resistant Graft Versus Host Disease: A Phase I, Multicenter, Open-Label, Dose-Escalation Study." *Nature Medicine* 26 (11): 1720-1725.

Bonab, Mandana Mohyeddin, Kamran Alimoghaddam, Fatemeh Talebian, Syed Hamid Ghaffari, Ardeshir Ghavamzadeh, and Behrouz Nikbin. 2006. "Aging of Mesenchymal Stem Cell in Vitro." *BMC Cell Biology* 7 (1): 1-7.

Bravery, Christopher A. 2015. "Do Human Leukocyte Antigen-Typed Cellular Therapeutics Based on Induced Pluripotent Stem Cells make Commercial Sense?" *Stem Cells and Development* 24 (1): 1-10.

Bruyneel, Arne A.N., Wesley L. McKeithan, Dries A.M. Feyen, and Mark Mercola. 2018. "Will iPSC-Cardiomyocytes Revolutionize the Discovery of Drugs for Heart Disease?" *Current Opinion in Pharmacology* 42: 55-61.

Butt, Sheraz A., Jørgen L. Jeppesen, Christian Torp-Pedersen, Flora Sam, Gunnar H. Gislason, Søren Jacobsen, and Charlotte Andersson. 2019. "Cardiovascular Manifestations of Systemic Sclerosis: A Danish Nationwide Cohort Study." *Journal of the American Heart Association* 8 (17): e013405.

Carvajal-Vergara, Xonia, Ana Sevilla, Sunita L. D'Souza, Yen-Sin Ang, Christoph Schaniel, Dung-Fang Lee, Lei Yang, Aaron D. Kaplan, Eric D. Adler, and Roye Rozov. 2010. "Patient-Specific Induced Pluripotent Stem-Cell-Derived Models of LEOPARD Syndrome." *Nature* 465 (7299): 808-812.

Champion, Hunter C. 2008. "The Heart in Scleroderma." *Rheumatic Disease Clinics of North America* 34 (1): 181-190.

Chen, Kevin G., Barbara S. Mallon, Rebecca S. Hamilton, Olga A. Kozhich, Kyeyoon Park, Daniel J. Hoeppner, Pamela G. Robey, and Ronald DG McKay. 2012. "Non-Colony Type Monolayer Culture of Human Embryonic Stem Cells." *Stem Cell Research* 9 (3): 237-248.

Chen, Shao-liang, Wu-wang Fang, Fei Ye, Yu-Hao Liu, Jun Qian, Shou-jie Shan, Jun-jie Zhang, Robert Zhao Chunhua, Lian-ming Liao, and Song Lin. 2004. "Effect on Left Ventricular Function of Intracoronary Transplantation of Autologous Bone Marrow Mesenchymal Stem Cell in Patients with Acute Myocardial Infarction." *The American Journal of Cardiology* 94 (1): 92-95.

Chimenti, Isotta, Rachel Ruckdeschel Smith, Tao-Sheng Li, Gary Gerstenblith, Elisa Messina, Alessandro Giacomello, and Eduardo Marbán. 2010. "Novelty and Significance." *Circulation Research* 106 (5): 971-980.

Chiossone, Laura, Romana Conte, Grazia Maria Spaggiari, Martina Serra, Cristina Romei, Francesca Bellora, Flavio Becchetti, Antonio Andaloro, Lorenzo Moretta, and Cristina Bottino. 2016. "Mesenchymal Stromal Cells Induce Peculiar Alternatively Activated Macrophages Capable of Dampening both Innate and Adaptive Immune Responses." *Stem Cells* 34 (7): 1909-1921.

Chong, James J.H., Xiulan Yang, Creighton W. Don, Elina Minami, Yen-Wen Liu, Jill J. Weyers, William M. Mahoney, Benjamin Van Biber, Savannah M. Cook, and Nathan J. Palpant. 2014. "Human Embryonic-Stem-Cell-Derived Cardiomyocytes Regenerate Non-Human Primate Hearts." *Nature* 510 (7504): 273-277.

Chu, Axel J., Eric Jiahua Zhao, Mu Chiao, and Chinten James Lim. 2020. "Co-Culture of Induced Pluripotent Stem Cells with Cardiomyocytes is Sufficient to Promote their Differentiation into Cardiomyocytes." *PloS One* 15 (4): e0230966.

Constantinou, Chrystalla, Antonio MA Miranda, Patricia Chaves, Mohamed Bellahcene, Andrea Massaia, Kevin Cheng, Sara Samari, Stephen M. Rothery, Anita M. Chandler, and Richard P. Schwarz. 2020. "Human Pluripotent Stem Cell-Derived Cardiomyocytes as a Target Platform for Paracrine Protection by Cardiac Mesenchymal Stromal Cells." *Scientific Reports* 10 (1): 1-18.

Crisan, Mihaela, Solomon Yap, Louis Casteilla, Chien-Wen Chen, Mirko Corselli, Tea Soon Park, Gabriella Andriolo, Bin Sun, Bo Zheng, and Li Zhang. 2008. "A Perivascular Origin for Mesenchymal Stem Cells in Multiple Human Organs." *Cell Stem Cell* 3 (3): 301-313.

Cyranoski, David. 2018. "'Reprogrammed'Stem Cells Approved to Mend Human Hearts for the First Time." *Nature* 557 (7706): 619.

Daley, Jim. 2018. "World's First Commercial iPSC Cell Plant Opens in Japan." *Japan Pharmaceutical*, Mar 23, 1. https://www.the-scientist.com/the-nutshell/worlds-first-commercial-ipsc-cell-plant-opens-in-japan-29915.

Davis, Darryl R., Rachel Ruckdeschel Smith, and Eduardo Marbán. 2010. "Human Cardiospheres are a Source of Stem Cells with Cardiomyo-genic Potential." *Stem Cells (Dayton, Ohio)* 28 (5): 903.

de Almeida, Danilo Candido, Marcelo RP Ferreira, Julia Franzen, Carola I. Weidner, Joana Frobel, Martin Zenke, Ivan G. Costa, and Wolfgang Wagner. 2016. "Epigenetic Classification of Human Mesenchymal Stromal Cells." *Stem Cell Reports* 6 (2): 168-175.

Devito, Liani, Anastasia Petrova, Cristian Miere, Stefano Codognotto, Nicola Blakely, Archie Lovatt, Caroline Ogilvie, Yacoub Khalaf, and Dusko Ilic. 2014. "Cost-effective Master Cell Bank Validation of Multiple Clinical-grade Human Pluripotent Stem Cell Lines from a Single Donor." *Stem Cells Translational Medicine* 3 (10): 1116-1124.

Di Baldassarre, Angela, Elisa Cimetta, Sveva Bollini, Giulia Gaggi, and Barbara Ghinassi. 2018. "Human-Induced Pluripotent Stem Cell Technology and Cardiomyocyte Generation: Progress and Clinical Applications." *Cells* 7 (6): 48.

Duelen, Robin and Maurilio Sampaolesi. 2017. "Stem Cell Technology in Cardiac Regeneration: A Pluripotent Stem Cell Promise." *EBioMedicine* 16: 30-40.

Emani, Sitaram M. and Pedro J. Del Nido. 2018. "No Title." *Cell-Based Therapy with Cardiosphere-Derived Cardiocytes: A New Hope for Pediatric Patients with Single Ventricle Congenital Heart Disease?*.

Eschenhagen, Thomas, Roberto Bolli, Thomas Braun, Loren J. Field, Bernd K. Fleischmann, Jonas Frisén, Mauro Giacca, Joshua M. Hare, Steven Houser, and Richard T. Lee. 2017. "Cardiomyocyte Regeneration: A Consensus Statement." *Circulation* 136 (7): 680-686.

Fukuda, Keiichi. 2001. "Development of Regenerative Cardiomyocytes from Mesenchymal Stem Cells for Cardiovascular Tissue Engineering." *Artificial Organs* 25 (3): 187-193.

Garbutt, Tiffany A., Jiandong Liu, and Li Qian. 2020. "Heart Regeneration using Somatic Cells." In *Emerging Technologies for Heart Diseases*, 259-283: Elsevier.

Gintant, Gary, Paul Burridge, Lior Gepstein, Sian Harding, Todd Herron, Charles Hong, José Jalife, Joseph C. Wu, and American Heart Association Council on Basic Cardiovascular Sciences. 2019. "Use of Human Induced Pluripotent Stem Cell–Derived Cardiomyocytes in Preclinical Cancer Drug Cardiotoxicity Testing: A Scientific Statement from the American Heart Association." *Circulation Research* 125 (10): e75-e92.

Guo, Jun, Guo-sheng Lin, Cui-yu Bao, Zhi-min Hu, and Ming-yan Hu. 2007. "Anti-Inflammation Role for Mesenchymal Stem Cells Transplantation in Myocardial Infarction." *Inflammation* 30 (3-4): 97-104.

Guo, Yajun, Yunsheng Yu, Shijun Hu, Yueqiu Chen, and Zhenya Shen. 2020. "The Therapeutic Potential of Mesenchymal Stem Cells for Cardiovascular Diseases." *Cell Death & Disease* 11 (5): 1-10.

Hare, Joshua M., Joel E. Fishman, Gary Gerstenblith, Darcy L. DiFede Velazquez, Juan P. Zambrano, Viky Y. Suncion, Melissa Tracy, Eduard Ghersin, Peter V. Johnston, and Jeffrey A. Brinker. 2012. "Comparison of Allogeneic Vs Autologous Bone Marrow–derived Mesenchymal Stem Cells Delivered by Transendocardial Injection in Patients with Ischemic Cardiomyopathy: The POSEIDON Randomized Trial." *Jama* 308 (22): 2369-2379.

Hare, Joshua M., Jay H. Traverse, Timothy D. Henry, Nabil Dib, Robert K. Strumpf, Steven P. Schulman, Gary Gerstenblith, Anthony N. DeMaria, Ali E. Denktas, and Roger S. Gammon. 2009. "A Randomized, Double-Blind, Placebo-Controlled, Dose-Escalation Study of Intravenous Adult Human Mesenchymal Stem Cells (Prochymal) After Acute Myocardial Infarction." *Journal of the American College of Cardiology* 54 (24): 2277-2286.

Hinson, John T., Anant Chopra, Navid Nafissi, William J. Polacheck, Craig C. Benson, Sandra Swist, Joshua Gorham, Luhan Yang, Sebastian Schafer, and

Calvin C. Sheng. 2015. "Titin Mutations in iPS Cells Define Sarcomere Insufficiency as a Cause of Dilated Cardiomy-opathy." *Science* 349 (6251): 982-986.

Hirt, Marc N., Jasper Boeddinghaus, Alice Mitchell, Sebastian Schaaf, Christian Börnchen, Christian Müller, Herbert Schulz, Norbert Hubner, Justus Stenzig, and Andrea Stoehr. 2014. "Functional Improvement and Maturation of Rat and Human Engineered Heart Tissue by Chronic Electrical Stimulation." *Journal of Molecular and Cellular Cardiology* 74: 151-161.

Horwitz, Edwin M., Patricia L. Gordon, Winston KK Koo, Jeffrey C. Marx, Michael D. Neel, Rene Y. McNall, Linda Muul, and Ted Hofmann. 2002. "Isolated Allogeneic Bone Marrow-Derived Mesenchymal Cells Engraft and Stimulate Growth in Children with Osteogenesis Imperfecta: Implications for Cell Therapy of Bone." *Proceedings of the National Academy of Sciences* 99 (13): 8932-8937.

Horwitz, Edwin M., Darwin J. Prockop, Patricia L. Gordon, Winston WK Koo, Lorraine A. Fitzpatrick, Michael D. Neel, M. Elizabeth McCarville, Paul J. Orchard, Reed E. Pyeritz, and Malcolm K. Brenner. 2001. "Clinical Responses to Bone Marrow Transplantation in Children with Severe Osteogenesis Imperfecta." *Blood, the Journal of the American Society of Hematology* 97 (5): 1227-1231.

Huang, Ching-Ying, Chun-Lin Liu, Chien-Yu Ting, Yueh-Ting Chiu, Yu-Che Cheng, Martin W. Nicholson, and Patrick CH Hsieh. 2019. "Human iPSC Banking: Barriers and Opportunities." *Journal of Biomedical Science* 26 (1): 1-14.

Huang, Ngan F., Vahid Serpooshan, Viola B. Morris, Nazish Sayed, Gaspard Pardon, Oscar J. Abilez, Karina H. Nakayama, Beth L. Pruitt, Sean M. Wu, and Young-sup Yoon. 2018. "Big Bottlenecks in Cardiovascular Tissue Engineering." *Communications Biology* 1 (1): 1-4.

Huang, Xiaowu, Huanhuan Wang, and Yong Xu. 2020. "Induced Pluripotent Stem Cells (iPSC)-Derived Mesenchymal Stem Cells (MSCs) showed Comparable Effects in Repair of Acute Kidney Injury as Compared to Adult MSCs." *Urology Journal* 17 (2): 204-209.

Ilic, Dusko. 2016. "No Title." *iPSC in the Past Decade: The Japanese Dominance.*

Insausti, Carmen L., Miguel Blanquer, Ana M. García-Hernández, Gregorio Castellanos, and José M. Moraleda. 2014. "Amniotic Membrane-Derived Stem Cells: Immunomodulatory Properties and Potential Clinical Application." *Stem Cells and Cloning: Advances and Applications* 7: 53.

Itskovitz-Eldor, Joseph, Maya Schuldiner, Dorit Karsenti, Amir Eden, Ofra Yanuka, Michal Amit, Hermona Soreq, and Nissim Benvenisty. 2000. "Differentiation of Human Embryonic Stem Cells into Embryoid Bodies

Comprising the Three Embryonic Germ Layers." *Molecular Medicine* 6 (2): 88-95.

Ji, Wanqing, Bo Hou, Weige Lin, Linli Wang, Wenhan Zheng, Weidong Li, Jie Zheng, Xuejun Wen, and Ping He. 2020. "3D Bioprinting a Human iPSC-Derived MSC-Loaded Scaffold for Repair of the Uterine Endometrium." *Acta Biomaterialia* 116: 268-284.

Jin, Bo, Xinping Luo, Haihong Lin, Jian Li, and Haiming Shi. 2010. "A Meta-analysis of Erythropoiesis-stimulating Agents in Anaemic Patients with Chronic Heart Failure." *European Journal of Heart Failure* 12 (3): 249-253.

Johnston, Peter V., Tetsuo Sasano, Kevin Mills, Robert Evers, Shuo-Tsan Lee, Rachel Ruckdeschel Smith, Albert C. Lardo, Shenghan Lai, Charles Steenbergen, and Gary Gerstenblith. 2009. "Clinical Perspective." *Circulation* 120 (12): 1075-1083.

Karantalis, Vasileios, Darcy L. DiFede, Gary Gerstenblith, Si Pham, James Symes, Juan Pablo Zambrano, Joel Fishman, Pradip Pattany, Ian McNiece, and John Conte. 2014. "Autologous Mesenchymal Stem Cells Produce Concordant Improvements in Regional Function, Tissue Perfusion, and Fibrotic Burden when Administered to Patients Undergoing Coronary Artery Bypass Grafting: The Prospective Randomized Study of Mesenchymal Stem Cell Therapy in Patients Undergoing Cardiac Surgery (PROMETHEUS) Trial." *Circulation Research* 114 (8): 1302-1310.

Kassem, Moustapha. 2004. "Mesenchymal Stem Cells: Biological Characteristics and Potential Clinical Applications." *Cloning and Stem Cells* 6 (4): 369-374.

Katritsis, Demosthenes G., Panagiota Sotiropoulou, Eleftherios Giazitzoglou, Evangelia Karvouni, and Michael Papamichail. 2007. "Electrophysiological Effects of Intracoronary Transplantation of Autologous Mesenchymal and Endothelial Progenitor Cells." *Europace* 9 (3): 167-171.

Khan, Mohammad Afzal, Fatimah Alanazi, Hala Abdalrahman Ahmed, Talal Shamma, Kilian Kelly, Mohamed A. Hammad, Abdullah O. Alawad, Abdullah Mohammed Assiri, and Dieter Clemens Broering. 2019. "iPSC-Derived MSC Therapy Induces Immune Tolerance and Supports Long-Term Graft Survival in Mouse Orthotopic Tracheal Transplants." *Stem Cell Research & Therapy* 10 (1): 1-15.

Kilpinen, Helena, Angela Goncalves, Andreas Leha, Vackar Afzal, Kaur Alasoo, Sofie Ashford, Sendu Bala, Dalila Bensaddek, Francesco Paolo Casale, and Oliver J. Culley. 2017. "Common Genetic Variation Drives Molecular Heterogeneity in Human iPSCs." *Nature* 546 (7658): 370-375.

Kobayashi, Kazuya and Ken Suzuki. 2018. "Mesenchymal Stem/Stromal Cell-Based Therapy for Heart Failure—What is the Best Source?" *Circulation Journal* 82 (9): 2222-2232.

Koç, Omer N., Stanton L. Gerson, Brenda W. Cooper, Stephanie M. Dyhouse, Stephen E. Haynesworth, Arnold I. Caplan, and Hillard M. Lazarus. 2000. "Rapid Hematopoietic Recovery After Coinfusion of Autologous-Blood Stem Cells and Culture-Expanded Marrow Mesenchymal Stem Cells in Advanced Breast Cancer Patients Receiving High-Dose Chemotherapy." *Journal of Clinical Oncology* 18 (2): 307.

Kucia, Magda, Buddhadeb Dawn, Greg Hunt, Yiru Guo, Marcin Wysoczynski, Marcin Majka, Janina Ratajczak, Francine Rezzoug, Suzanne T. Ildstad, and Roberto Bolli. 2004. "Cells Expressing Early Cardiac Markers Reside in the Bone Marrow and are Mobilized into the Peripheral Blood After Myocardial Infarction." *Circulation Research* 95 (12): 1191-1199.

Laflamme, Michael A. and Charles E. Murry. 2005. "Regenerating the Heart." *Nature Biotechnology* 23 (7): 845-856.

Lázár, Enikő, Hesham A. Sadek, and Olaf Bergmann. 2017. "Cardiomyo-cyte Renewal in the Human Heart: Insights from the Fall-Out." *European Heart Journal* 38 (30): 2333-2342.

Lazarus, HillardM, S. E. Haynesworth, S. L. Gerson, N. S. Rosenthal, and A. I. Caplan. 1995. "Ex Vivo Expansion and Subsequent Infusion of Human Bone Marrow-Derived Stromal Progenitor Cells (Mesenchymal Progenitor Cells): Implications for Therapeutic use." *Bone Marrow Transplantation* 16 (4): 557-564.

Le, TYL and J.J.H. Chong. 2016. "Cardiac Progenitor Cells for Heart Repair." *Cell Death Discovery* 2 (1): 1-4.

Ledesma-Martínez, Edgar, Víctor Manuel Mendoza-Núñez, and Edelmiro Santiago-Osorio. 2016. "Mesenchymal Stem Cells Derived from Dental Pulp: A Review." *Stem Cells International* 2016.

Lee, Jun-Won, Seung-Hwan Lee, Young-Jin Youn, Min-Soo Ahn, Jang-Young Kim, Byung-Su Yoo, Junghan Yoon, Woocheol Kwon, In-Soo Hong, and Kyounghoon Lee. 2014. "A Randomized, Open-Label, Multicenter Trial for the Safety and Efficacy of Adult Mesenchymal Stem Cells after Acute Myocardial Infarction." *Journal of Korean Medical Science* 29 (1): 23.

Leppo, Michelle K., Joshua M. Hare, Elisa Messina, Alessandro Giacomello, M. Roselle Abraham, and Eduardo Marbán. 2007. "Regenerative Potential of Cardiosphere-Derived Cells Expanded from Percutaneous Endomyocardial Biopsy Specimens." *Circulation*.

Li, Junjun, Ying Hua, Shigeru Miyagawa, Jingbo Zhang, Lingjun Li, Li Liu, and Yoshiki Sawa. 2020. "hiPSC-Derived Cardiac Tissue for Disease Modeling and Drug Discovery." *International Journal of Molecular Sciences* 21 (23): 8893.

Li, Tao-Sheng, Ke Cheng, Shuo-Tsan Lee, Satoshi Matsushita, Darryl Davis, Konstantinos Malliaras, Yiqiang Zhang, Noriko Matsushita, Rachel

Ruckdeschel Smith, and Eduardo Marbán. 2010. "Cardiospheres Recapitulate a Niche-like Microenvironment Rich in Stemness and Cell-matrix Interactions, Rationalizing their Enhanced Functional Potency for Myocardial Repair." *Stem Cells* 28 (11): 2088-2098.

Li, Tao-Sheng, Ke Cheng, Konstantinos Malliaras, Rachel Ruckdeschel Smith, Yiqiang Zhang, Baiming Sun, Noriko Matsushita, Agnieszka Blusztajn, John Terrovitis, and Hideo Kusuoka. 2012. "Direct Comparison of Different Stem Cell Types and Subpopulations Reveals Superior Paracrine Potency and Myocardial Repair Efficacy with Cardiosphere-Derived Cells." *Journal of the American College of Cardiology* 59 (10): 942-953.

Lian, Xiaojun, Cheston Hsiao, Gisela Wilson, Kexian Zhu, Laurie B. Hazeltine, Samira M. Azarin, Kunil K. Raval, Jianhua Zhang, Timothy J. Kamp, and Sean P. Palecek. 2012. "Robust Cardiomyocyte Differentiation from Human Pluripotent Stem Cells via Temporal Modulation of Canonical Wnt Signaling." *Proceedings of the National Academy of Sciences* 109 (27): E1848-E1857.

Lian, Xiaojun, Jianhua Zhang, Samira M. Azarin, Kexian Zhu, Laurie B. Hazeltine, Xiaoping Bao, Cheston Hsiao, Timothy J. Kamp, and Sean P. Palecek. 2013. "Directed Cardiomyocyte Differentiation from Human Pluripotent Stem Cells by Modulating Wnt/B-Catenin Signaling Under Fully Defined Conditions." *Nature Protocols* 8 (1): 162-175.

Liaw, Norman Yu and Wolfram-Hubertus Zimmermann. 2016. "Mechani-cal Stimulation in the Engineering of Heart Muscle." *Advanced Drug Delivery Reviews* 96: 156-160.

Liu, Jingbo, Qingsong Hu, Zongli Wang, Chengsu Xu, Xiaohong Wang, Guangrong Gong, Abdul Mansoor, Joseph Lee, Mingxiao Hou, and Lepeng Zeng. 2004. "Autologous Stem Cell Transplantation for Myocardial Repair." *American Journal of Physiology-Heart and Circulatory Physiology* 287 (2): H501-H511.

Liu, Yen-Wen, Billy Chen, Xiulan Yang, James A. Fugate, Faith A. Kalucki, Akiko Futakuchi-Tsuchida, Larry Couture, Keith W. Vogel, Clifford A. Astley, and Audrey Baldessari. 2018. "Human Embryonic Stem Cell–derived Cardiomyocytes Restore Function in Infarcted Hearts of Non-Human Primates." *Nature Biotechnology* 36 (7): 597-605.

Lu, Lei, Min Liu, RongRong Sun, Yi Zheng, and Peiying Zhang. 2015. "Myocardial Infarction: Symptoms and Treatments." *Cell Biochemistry and Biophysics* 72 (3): 865-867.

Lundy, Scott D., Wei-Zhong Zhu, Michael Regnier, and Michael A. Laflamme. 2013. "Structural and Functional Maturation of Cardiomyocytes Derived from Human Pluripotent Stem Cells." *Stem Cells and Development* 22 (14): 1991-2002.

Machiraju, Pranav and Steven C. Greenway. 2019. "Current Methods for the Maturation of Induced Pluripotent Stem Cell-Derived Cardiomyocytes." *World Journal of Stem Cells* 11 (1): 33.

Makino, Shinji, Keiichi Fukuda, Shunichirou Miyoshi, Fusako Konishi, Hiroaki Kodama, Jing Pan, Motoaki Sano, Toshiyuki Takahashi, Shingo Hori, and Hitoshi Abe. 1999. "Cardiomyocytes can be Generated from Marrow Stromal Cells in Vitro." *The Journal of Clinical Investigation* 103 (5): 697-705.

Makkar, Raj R., Rachel R. Smith, K. E. Cheng, Konstantinos Malliaras, Louise E.J. Thomson, Daniel Berman, Lawrence S.C. Czer, Linda Marbán, Adam Mendizabal, and Peter V. Johnston. 2012. "Intracoronary Cardiosphere-Derived Cells for Heart Regeneration after Myocardial Infarction (CADUCEUS): A Prospective, Randomised Phase 1 Trial." *The Lancet* 379 (9819): 895-904.

Malliaras, Konstantinos, Raj R. Makkar, Rachel R. Smith, Ke Cheng, Edwin Wu, Robert O. Bonow, Linda Marbán, Adam Mendizabal, Eugenio Cingolani, and Peter V. Johnston. 2014. "Intracoronary Cardiosphere-Derived Cells after Myocardial Infarction: Evidence of Therapeutic Regeneration in the Final 1-Year Results of the CADUCEUS Trial (CArdiosphere-Derived aUtologous Stem CElls to Reverse ventricUlar dySfunction)." *Journal of the American College of Cardiology* 63 (2): 110-122.

Martin, Ulrich. 2017. "Genome Stability of Programmed Stem Cell Products." *Advanced Drug Delivery Reviews* 120: 108-117.

Matsa, Elena, Divya Rajamohan, Emily Dick, Lorraine Young, Ian Mellor, Andrew Staniforth, and Chris Denning. 2011. "Drug Evaluation in Cardiomyocytes Derived from Human Induced Pluripotent Stem Cells Carrying a Long QT Syndrome Type 2 Mutation." *European Heart Journal* 32 (8): 952-962.

Mazzola, Marta and Elisa Di Pasquale. 2020. "Toward Cardiac Regeneration: Combination of Pluripotent Stem Cell-Based Therapies and Bioengineering Strategies." *Frontiers in Bioengineering and Biotechnology* 8.

Menasché, Philippe. 2015. "Stem Cells for the Treatment of Heart Failure." *Philosophical Transactions of the Royal Society B: Biologi-cal Sciences* 370 (1680): 20140373.

Messina, Elisa, Luciana De Angelis, Giacomo Frati, Stefania Morrone, Stefano Chimenti, Fabio Fiordaliso, Monica Salio, Massimo Battaglia, Michael VG Latronico, and Marcello Coletta. 2004. "Isolation and Expansion of Adult Cardiac Stem Cells from Human and Murine Heart." *Circulation Research* 95 (9): 911-921.

Miao, Qingfeng, Winston Shim, Nicole Tee, Sze Yun Lim, Ying Ying Chung, K.P. Myu Mia Ja, Ting Huay Ooi, Grace Tan, Geraldine Kong, and Heming Wei. 2014. "iPSC-derived Human Mesenchymal Stem Cells Improve

Myocardial Strain of Infarcted Myocardium." *Journal of Cellular and Molecular Medicine* 18 (8): 1644-1654.

Mirotsou, Maria, Tilanthi M. Jayawardena, Jeffrey Schmeckpeper, Massimiliano Gnecchi, and Victor J. Dzau. 2011. "Paracrine Mechanisms of Stem Cell Reparative and Regenerative Actions in the Heart." *Journal of Molecular and Cellular Cardiology* 50 (2): 280-289.

Mohy, Aldin Bonab M., B. Nikbin, Hassani Mr Mohamad, Mehdi Sanatkar, Masuod Gasemi, Hamid Mirkhani, Hassan Radmehr, Mehrdad Salehi, Massoud Eslami, and Parsa A. Farhig. 2007. "Autologous in Vitro Expanded Mesenchymal Stem Cell Therapy for Human Old Myocardial Infarction."

Mokino, S. and K. Fududa. 1999. "Miyoshi Set a/. Cardiomyocyte can be Generated from Marrow Stromal Cell in Vitro." *J Clin Invest I* 999: 103.

Moradi, Sharif, Hamid Mahdizadeh, Tomo Šarić, Johnny Kim, Javad Harati, Hosein Shahsavarani, Boris Greber, and Joseph B. Moore. 2019. "Research and Therapy with Induced Pluripotent Stem Cells (iPSCs): Social, Legal, and Ethical Considerations." *Stem Cell Research & Therapy* 10 (1): 1-13.

Mukherjee, Monica, Sanjiv Shah, John Varga, and Susan B. Yeon. *Cardiac Manifestations of Systemic Sclerosis (Scleroderma).*

Müller, Paula, Heiko Lemcke, and Robert David. 2018. "Stem Cell Therapy in Heart Diseases–cell Types, Mechanisms and Improvement Strategies." *Cellular Physiology and Biochemistry* 48 (6): 2607-2655.

Mummery, Christine L., Jianhua Zhang, Elizabeth S. Ng, David A. Elliott, Andrew G. Elefanty, and Timothy J. Kamp. 2012. "Differentiation of Human Embryonic Stem Cells and Induced Pluripotent Stem Cells to Cardiomyocytes: A Methods Overview." *Circulation Research* 111 (3): 344-358.

Musiał-Wysocka, Aleksandra, Marta Kot, and Marcin Majka. 2019. "The Pros and Cons of Mesenchymal Stem Cell-Based Therapies." *Cell Transplantation* 28 (7): 801-812.

Najar, Mehdi, Gordana Raicevic, Hussein Fayyad-Kazan, Dominique Bron, Michel Toungouz, and Laurence Lagneaux. 2016. "Mesenchy-mal Stromal Cells and Immunomodulation: A Gathering of Regulatory Immune Cells." *Cytotherapy* 18 (2): 160-171.

Nartprayut, Kuneerat, Pakpoom Kheolamai, Sirikul Manochantr, Methichit Chayosumrit, Surapol Issaragrisil, and Aungkura Supokawej. 2013. "Cardiomyocyte Differentiation of Perinatally-derived Mesenchymal Stem Cells." *Molecular Medicine Reports* 7 (5): 1465-1469.

Neofytou, Evgenios, Connor Galen O'Brien, Larry A. Couture, and Joseph C. Wu. 2015. "Hurdles to Clinical Translation of Human Induced Pluripotent Stem Cells." *The Journal of Clinical Investigation* 125 (7): 2551-2557.

Nguyen, Doan C., Tracy A. Hookway, Qingling Wu, Rajneesh Jha, Marcela K. Preininger, Xuemin Chen, Charles A. Easley, Paul Spearman, Shriprasad R. Deshpande, and Kevin Maher. 2014. "Microscale Generation of Cardiospheres Promotes Robust Enrichment of Cardiomyocytes Derived from Human Pluripotent Stem Cells." *Stem Cell Reports* 3 (2): 260-268.

NIH U.S. National Library of Medicine. *ClinicalTrials.Gov.*, clinicaltrials.gov.

Ohnishi, Shunsuke, Bobby Yanagawa, Koichi Tanaka, Yoshinori Miyahara, Hiroaki Obata, Masaharu Kataoka, Makoto Kodama, Hatsue Ishibashi-Ueda, Kenji Kangawa, and Soichiro Kitamura. 2007. "Transplantation of Mesenchymal Stem Cells Attenuates Myocardial Injury and Dysfunction in a Rat Model of Acute Myocarditis." *Journal of Molecular and Cellular Cardiology* 42 (1): 88-97.

Oikonomopoulos, Angelos, Tomoya Kitani, and Joseph C. Wu. 2018. "Pluripotent Stem Cell-Derived Cardiomyocytes as a Platform for Cell Therapy Applications: Progress and Hurdles for Clinical Translation." *Molecular Therapy* 26 (7): 1624-1634.

Parekkadan, Biju and Jack M. Milwid. 2010. "Mesenchymal Stem Cells as Therapeutics." *Annual Review of Biomedical Engineering* 12: 87-117.

Park, Misun and Young-sup Yoon. 2018. "Cardiac Regeneration with Human Pluripotent Stem Cell-Derived Cardiomyocytes." *Korean Circulation Journal* 48 (11): 974.

Parrotta, Elvira Immacolata, Valeria Lucchino, Luana Scaramuzzino, Stefania Scalise, and Giovanni Cuda. 2020. "Modeling Cardiac Disease Mechanisms using Induced Pluripotent Stem Cell-Derived Cardiomyocytes: Progress, Promises and Challenges." *International Journal of Molecular Sciences* 21 (12): 4354.

Pettinato, Giuseppe, Xuejun Wen, and Ning Zhang. 2015. "Engineering Strategies for the Formation of Embryoid Bodies from Human Pluripotent Stem Cells." *Stem Cells and Development* 24 (14): 1595-1609.

Pittenger, Mark F., Dennis E. Discher, Bruno M. Péault, Donald G. Phinney, Joshua M. Hare, and Arnold I. Caplan. 2019. "Mesenchymal Stem Cell Perspective: Cell Biology to Clinical Progress." *NPJ Regenerative Medicine* 4 (1): 1-15.

Pittenger, Mark F., Alastair M. Mackay, Stephen C. Beck, Rama K. Jaiswal, Robin Douglas, Joseph D. Mosca, Mark A. Moorman, Donald W. Simonetti, Stewart Craig, and Daniel R. Marshak. 1999. "Multilineage Potential of Adult Human Mesenchymal Stem Cells." *Science* 284 (5411): 143-147.

Prescott, Catherine. 2011. "The Business of Exploiting Induced Pluripotent Stem Cells." *Philosophical Transactions of the Royal Society B: Biological Sciences* 366 (1575): 2323-2328.

Robinton, Daisy A. and George Q. Daley. 2012. "The Promise of Induced Pluripotent Stem Cells in Research and Therapy." *Nature* 481 (7381): 295-305.

Røsland, Gro Vatne, Agnete Svendsen, Anja Torsvik, Ewa Sobala, Emmet McCormack, Heike Immervoll, Josef Mysliwietz, Joerg-Christian Tonn, Roland Goldbrunner, and Per Eystein Lønning. 2009. "Long-Term Cultures of Bone Marrow–derived Human Mesenchymal Stem Cells Frequently Undergo Spontaneous Malignant Transformation." *Cancer Research* 69 (13): 5331-5339.

Sachs, Patrick C., Michael P. Francis, Min Zhao, Jenni Brumelle, Raj R. Rao, Lynne W. Elmore, and Shawn E. Holt. 2012. "Defining Essential Stem Cell Characteristics in Adipose-Derived Stromal Cells Extracted from Distinct Anatomical Sites." *Cell and Tissue Research* 349 (2): 505-515.

Sambasiva Rao, K.R.S., K. Ananda Krishna, K. Sai Krishna, Ruben Berrocal, and K.S. Rao. "Myocardial Infarction and Stem Cells." *Journal of Pharmacy and Bioallied Sciences* 3 (2).

Segers, Vincent F.M. and Richard T. Lee. 2008. "Stem-Cell Therapy for Cardiac Disease." *Nature* 451 (7181): 937-942.

Senyo, Samuel E., Matthew L. Steinhauser, Christie L. Pizzimenti, Vicky K. Yang, Lei Cai, Mei Wang, Ting-Di Wu, Jean-Luc Guerquin-Kern, Claude P. Lechene, and Richard T. Lee. 2013. "Mammalian Heart Renewal by Pre-Existing Cardiomyocytes." *Nature* 493 (7432): 433-436.

Shi, Shutian, Xingxin Wu, Xiao Wang, Wen Hao, Huangtai Miao, Lei Zhen, and Shaoping Nie. 2016. "Differentiation of Bone Marrow Mesenchymal Stem Cells to Cardiomyocyte-Like Cells is Regulated by the Combined Low Dose Treatment of Transforming Growth Factor-B1 and 5-Azacytidine." *Stem Cells International* 2016.

Shokraei, Nasim, Shiva Asadpour, Shabnam Shokraei, Mehrdad Nasrollahzadeh Sabet, Reza Faridi-Majidi, and Hossein Ghanbari. 2019. "Development of Electrically Conductive Hybrid Nanofibers Based on CNT-polyurethane Nanocomposite for Cardiac Tissue Engineering." *Microscopy Research and Technique* 82 (8): 1316-1325.

Smith, Alec S.T., Jesse Macadangdang, Winnie Leung, Michael A. Laflamme, and Deok-Ho Kim. 2017. "Human iPSC-Derived Cardiomyocytes and Tissue Engineering Strategies for Disease Modeling and Drug Screening." *Biotechnology Advances* 35 (1): 77-94.

Souidi, Monia, Pascal Amédro, Pierre Meyer, Romain Desprat, Jean-Marc Lemaître, François Rivier, Alain Lacampagne, and Albano C. Meli. 2020. "Generation of Three Duchenne Muscular Dystrophy Patient-Specific Induced Pluripotent Stem Cell Lines DMD_YoTaz_PhyMedEXp,

DMD_RaPer_PhyMedEXp, DMD_OuMen_PhyMedEXp (INSRMi008-A, INSRMi009-A and INSRMi010-A)." *Stem Cell Research* 49: 102094.

Takahashi, Kazutoshi, Koji Tanabe, Mari Ohnuki, Megumi Narita, Tomoko Ichisaka, Kiichiro Tomoda, and Shinya Yamanaka. 2007. "Induction of Pluripotent Stem Cells from Adult Human Fibroblasts by Defined Factors." *Cell* 131 (5): 861-872.

Takahashi, Kazutoshi and Shinya Yamanaka. 2006. "Induction of Pluripotent Stem Cells from Mouse Embryonic and Adult Fibroblast Cultures by Defined Factors." *Cell* 126 (4): 663-676. doi:https://doi.org/10.1016 /j.cell.2006.07.024. https://www.sciencedirect.com/science/article/pii/ S009 2867406009767.

Talkhabi, Mahmood, Nasser Aghdami, and Hossein Baharvand. 2016. "Human Cardiomyocyte Generation from Pluripotent Stem Cells: A State-of-Art." *Life Sciences* 145: 98-113.

Tang, Bor Luen. 2020. "No Title." *Maturing Ipsc-Derived Cardiomyo-cytes.*

Tang, Yao Liang, Qiang Zhao, Y. Clare Zhang, Leilei Cheng, Mingya Liu, Jianhui Shi, Yin Zeng Yang, Chuizhen Pan, Junbo Ge, and M. Ian Phillips. 2004. "Autologous Mesenchymal Stem Cell Transplantation Induce VEGF and Neovascularization in Ischemic Myocardium." *Regulatory Peptides* 117 (1): 3-10.

Terashvili, Maia and Zeljko J. Bosnjak. 2019. "Stem Cell Therapies in Cardiovascular Disease." *Journal of Cardiothoracic and Vascular Anesthesia* 33 (1): 209-222.

Times, York. 2013. "Privacy and Protection in the Genomic Era." *Nature Medicine* 19 (9): 1073.

Turner, Darren, Angela C. Rieger, Wayne Balkan, and Joshua M. Hare. 2020. "Clinical-Based Cell Therapies for Heart Disease—Current and Future State." *Rambam Maimonides Medical Journal* 11 (2).

Ullah, Imran, Raghavendra Baregundi Subbarao, and Gyu Jin Rho. 2015. "Human Mesenchymal Stem Cells-Current Trends and Future Prospec-tive." *Bioscience Reports* 35 (2).

Vidarsson, Hilmar, Johan Hyllner, and Peter Sartipy. 2010. "Differenti-ation of Human Embryonic Stem Cells to Cardiomyocytes for in Vitro and in Vivo Applications." *Stem Cell Reviews and Reports* 6 (1): 108-120.

Wang, Deguo, Fengxiang Zhang, Wenzhi Shen, Minglong Chen, Bing Yang, Yuzhen Zhang, and Kejiang Cao. 2011. "Mesenchymal Stem Cell Injection Ameliorates the Inducibility of Ventricular Arrhythmias After Myocardial Infarction in Rats." *International Journal of Cardiology* 152 (3): 314-320. doi:https://doi.org/10.1016/j.ijcard.2010. 07.025. https://www.sciencedirect. com/science/article/pii/S0167527310005528.

Webster, R.A., S. P. Blaber, B.R. Herbert, M.R. Wilkins, and G. Vesey. 2012. "The Role of Mesenchymal Stem Cells in Veterinary Therapeutics–a Review." *New Zealand Veterinary Journal* 60 (5): 265-272.

White, Ian A., Cristina Sanina, Wayne Balkan, and Joshua M. Hare. 2016. "Mesenchymal Stem Cells in Cardiology." In *Mesenchymal Stem Cells*, 55-87: Springer.

Williams, Adam R., Barry Trachtenberg, Darcy L. Velazquez, Ian McNiece, Peter Altman, Didier Rouy, Adam M. Mendizabal, Pradip M. Pattany, Gustavo A. Lopera, and Joel Fishman. 2011. "Intramyo-cardial Stem Cell Injection in Patients with Ischemic Cardiomyopathy: Functional Recovery and Reverse Remodeling." *Circulation Research* 108 (7): 792-796.

World Health Organization, (WHO). 2020. "The Top 10 Causes of Death in 2019 Accounted for 55% of the World's Deaths: WHO." *CE Noticias Financieras*, Dec 9. https://search.proquest.com/docview/2469033428.

Xu, Maojia, Georgina Shaw, Mary Murphy, and Frank Barry. 2019. "Induced Pluripotent Stem Cell-Derived Mesenchymal Stromal Cells are Functionally and Genetically Different from Bone Marrow-Derived Mesenchymal Stromal Cells." *Stem Cells* 37 (6): 754-765.

Xu, Wenrong, Xiran Zhang, Hui Qian, Wei Zhu, Xiaochun Sun, Jiabo Hu, Hong Zhou, and Yongchang Chen. 2004. "Mesenchymal Stern Cells from Adult Human Bone Marrow Differentiate into a Cardiomyocyte Phenotype in Vitro." *Experimental Biology and Medicine* 229 (7): 623-631.

Yang, Xiulan, Marita Rodriguez, Lil Pabon, Karin A. Fischer, Hans Reinecke, Michael Regnier, Nathan J. Sniadecki, Hannele Ruohola-Baker, and Charles E. Murry. 2014. "Tri-Iodo-L-Thyronine Promotes the Maturation of Human Cardiomyocytes-Derived from Induced Pluripotent Stem Cells." *Journal of Molecular and Cellular Cardiology* 72: 296-304.

Yoon, Jihyun, Wan Joo Shim, Young Moo Ro, and Do-Sun Lim. 2005. "Transdifferentiation of Mesenchymal Stem Cells into Cardiomyocytes by Direct Cell-to-Cell Contact with Neonatal Cardiomyocyte but Not Adult Cardiomyocytes." *Annals of Hemato-logy* 84 (11): 715-721.

Zebrowski, David C., Robert Becker, and Felix B. Engel. 2016. "Towards Regenerating the Mammalian Heart: Challenges in Evaluating Experimentally Induced Adult Mammalian Cardiomyocyte Proliferation." *American Journal of Physiology-Heart and Circulatory Physiology* 310 (9): H1045-H1054.

Zhang, J., Wilson G.F., Soerens A.G., Koonce C.H., Yu J, Palecek S.P., Thomson J.A., Kamp T.J." 2009. Functional Cardiomyocytes Derived from Human Induced Pluripotent Stem Cells. *Circ Res* 104: e30-e41.

Zhang, Jianhua, Kunil K. Raval, Xiaojun Lian, Amanda M. Herman, Gisela F. Wilson, Matthew R. Barron, Junying Yu, Sean P. Palecek, James A.

Thomson, and Timothy J. Kamp. 2010. "No Title." *Matrix-Promoted Efficient Cardiac Differentiation of Human iPS and ES Cells.*

Zhang, Yuelin, Xiaoting Liang, Songyan Liao, Weixin Wang, Junwen Wang, Xiang Li, Yue Ding, Yingmin Liang, Fei Gao, and Mo Yang. 2015. "Potent Paracrine Effects of Human Induced Pluripotent Stem Cell-Derived Mesenchymal Stem Cells Attenuate Doxorubicin-Induced Cardiomyopathy." *Scientific Reports* 5 (1): 1-17.

Zomer, Helena D., Atanásio S. Vidane, Natalia N. Gonçalves, and Carlos E. Ambrósio. 2015. "Mesenchymal and Induced Pluripotent Stem Cells: General Insights and Clinical Perspectives." *Stem Cells and Cloning: Advances and Applications* 8: 125.

Chapter 3

Transcatheter Aortic Valve Implantation versus Sutureless Aortic Valve Replacement: Overview of the Recent Advancements in Cardiac Surgery

Mathieu Rheault-Henry[1], MD
and Rony Atoui[2,*], MD
[1]Northern Ontario School of Medicine, Sudbury, Ontario, Canada
[2]Division of Cardiac Surgery, Health Sciences North,
Northern Ontario School of Medicine, Sudbury, Ontario, Canada

Abstract

Aortic stenosis is the most common valvulopathy and a significant cause of morbidity and mortality in older adults. Surgical aortic valve replacement (SAVR) with sutured prostheses currently remains the gold standard of treatment for severe aortic stenosis. However, this operation may not be an option for selected patient populations. New developments in the field of cardiac surgery have led to the introduction of less invasive options for low to high-risk patients with aortic stenosis, or patients who are not candidates for surgical aortic valve replacement. As a result, transcatheter aortic valve implantation (TAVI) and sutureless aortic valve replacement (SU-AVR) have emerged as valuable alternatives to surgical aortic valve replacement with the aim of reducing invasiveness of surgical procedure, morbidity, and mortality. The aim of this review

* Corresponding Author's E-mail: rony.atoui@gmail.com.

In: Horizons in World Cardiovascular Research. Volume 22
Editor: Eleanor H. Bennington
ISBN: 978-1-68507-568-2

article is to compare outcomes of patients who underwent TAVI with those who underwent SU-AVR. Study end points will include short and long-term mortality, postoperative renal failure, postoperative stroke, major bleeding episodes, vascular complications, paravalvular leak (PVL), cardiopulmonary bypass time and the need for pacemaker insertion.

Keywords: aortic valve replacement, TAVI, sutureless valves, aortic stenosis

Introduction

Aortic valve stenosis is the most common valvular pathology with a prevalence of 2.8% in adults older than 75 years (Meco, Miceli, Montisci et al. 2018). It is typically caused by progressive calcification of the aortic valve leaflets or by a congenital malformation of the valve, known as a bicuspid aortic valve. Aortic stenosis is the most common cause of left ventricular outflow tract obstruction. Left untreated, it can result in severe complications such as heart failure, stroke, aortic aneurysm, and sudden cardiac death. Surgical aortic valve replacement (SAVR) has been the standard of care for patients with severe symptomatic aortic stenosis, most commonly done through median sternotomy. In this approach, a mechanical or bioprosthetic valve made of bovine or porcine pericardium is placed and sutured into the aortic annulus. Although surgical aortic valve replacement has been considered the gold standard of treatment for decades, recent advancements in cardiac surgery have introduced less invasive approaches to aortic valve replacement (AVR) with the aim of reducing mortality, morbidity and to offer patients ineligible for surgery with a curative option. In the past, patients with aortic stenosis where surgery was contraindicated could only be offered diuretics and balloon valvuloplasty. These interventions served only as a palliative treatment with no mortality benefits (Mahmaljy, Tawney and Young, 2017).

For patients ineligible for surgical aortic valve replacement, transcatheter aortic valve implantation (TAVI) emerged initially as a lifeline for high-risk surgical candidates who were refused surgery (Shinn, Altarabsheh, Deo et al. 2018; Leon, Smith, Mack et al. 2016; Thyregod, Steinbrüchel, Ihle et al. 2015). This excellent non-invasive option has shown very good hemodynamic and clinical outcomes for up to 5 years in high-risk or patients deemed inoperable (Kapadia, Leon, Makkar et al. 2015).

Since then, TAVI is now recommended in these patient populations (Class IIa, level of evidence B) and has now recently been explored as an option for low to intermediate-risk patients (Nishimura, Otto, Bonow et al. 2017). Similarly, sutureless aortic valve replacement (SU-AVR) has been an increasingly attractive option for AVR as it combines both a surgical and minimally invasive approach offering reduced cardiopulmonary bypass and aortic cross-clamp times, which are both significant contributors to postoperative morbidity and mortality (Fischlein, Pfeiffer, Pollari et al. 2015). Aortic valve replacement is indicated in a variety of patients as seen below (Mahmaljy, Tawney and Young, 2017; Nishimura, Otto, Bonow et al. 2017).

1. Severe high-gradient aortic stenosis with symptoms (class I recommendation, level B evidence)
2. Asymptomatic patients with severe aortic stenosis and left ventricular ejection fraction <50% (class I recommendation, level B evidence)
3. Severe aortic stenosis when undergoing other cardiac surgery (class I recommendation, level B evidence)
4. Asymptomatic severe aortic stenosis and low surgical risk (class IIa recommendation, level B evidence)
5. Symptomatic with low-flow/low-gradient severe aortic stenosis (class IIa recommendation, level B evidence)
6. Moderate aortic stenosis and undergoing other cardiac surgery (class IIa recommendation, level C evidence)

With the increasing use of transcatheter aortic valve implantation and the recent applications of sutureless aortic valve replacement, the spectrum of treatment for aortic valvulopathies has increased, leaving patients with more available options than ever. This chapter will focus on the advancements in aortic valve replacement, notably, transcatheter aortic valve implantation and the use of sutureless aortic valve technology in patients with aortic valve stenosis. Study end points will include comparison of in-hospital mortality, 30-day, 1-year and 2-year mortality, postoperative renal failure, postoperative stroke, major bleeding episodes, vascular complications, paravalvular leak (PVL), pacemaker implantation and cardiopulmonary bypass time between these two procedures.

Surgical Aortic Valve Replacement: Indications, Technique, and Outcomes

Surgical aortic valve replacement is the most commonly used approach for AVR and has outstanding short- and long-term outcomes (Brown, O'Brien, Wu et al. 2009). To this day, it remains the gold standard of operation for aortic valve disease. It is performed through median sternotomy with cardiopulmonary bypass, otherwise known as the heart-lung machine. During surgical AVR, the diseased valve leaflets are excised, the aortic annulus is debrided and a series of interrupted or continuous sutures are placed to insert a mechanical or biological valve (Spadaccio, Alkhamees, and Al-Attar, 2019). A key advantage of SAVR is the surgeon's ability to have direct access to the diseased valve. This allows for careful inspection of the valve, aortic root, aortic arch, and surrounding structures. Moreover, it provides an opportunity for the surgeon to completely excise the diseased leaflets and debride the annulus in a thorough manner to prevent paravalvular leak (Meco, Miceli, Montisci et al. 2018). Paravalvular leak is defined as the leaking of blood between the aorta and the newly replaced aortic valve. It is not commonly seen in SAVR, though it is a frequent complication of TAVI and may be observed in SU-AVR. Even the presence of mild PVL is associated with significant reductions in 5-year survival post-op (Mack, Leon, Smith et al. 2015). For this reason, great attention is paid to PVL post procedure, as it is a major factor in the long-term success of the AVR. Surgical aortic valve replacement via median sternotomy also allows the surgeon to perform other procedures concomitantly such as coronary artery bypass grafting (CABG) and replacement of the aorta due to calcification or aortic aneurysm. Moreover, SAVR reduces the risk of neurological events intra and post-procedure and remains the only option for patients with endocarditis or bicuspid aortic valve (Mack, Leon, Smith et al. 2015; Spadaccio, Alkhamees, and Al-Attar, 2019). The main complications of surgical AVR include bleeding, acute kidney injury, cardiogenic shock and new onset or worsening atrial fibrillation (Thyregod, Steinbrüchel, Ihle et al. 2015). Major life-threatening complications are rare occurrences in SAVR. Patients with comorbidities such as unstable coronary syndromes, arrhythmias, lung disease, renal insufficiency, and decompensated heart failure are deemed high risk for surgery and may be unfit for SAVR. Some contraindications to aortic valve replacement include patients with a life expectancy of less than 12 months, myocardial infarction within the last 30 days, hypertrophic cardiomyopathy, left ventricular ejection fraction < 20%, pulmonary hypertension, end-stage kidney disease, stroke, or transient ischemic attack within the last 6 months (Wilson, McNabney, Weir-McCall et al. 2019). Moreover, SAVR may also be contraindicated in patients who have high risk of intraoperative challenges due to anatomical features such as a porcelain aorta, small aortic annulus, or history of radiation to the chest (Spadaccio, Alkhamees, and Al-Attar, 2019). These challenges have encouraged innovations in the field of cardiac surgery, resulting in the development of alternatives to SAVR in the form of transcatheter aortic valve implantation and sutureless aortic valve replacement as patients still require effective treatments.

Sutureless Aortic Valve Replacement: Indications, Technique, and Outcomes

While SAVR still represents the standard of care in the treatment of aortic stenosis, SU-AVR does not require anchoring sutures in the aortic annulus, yet still allows for complete excision of the diseased leaflets and debridement of the aortic annulus. This ultimately results in decreased aortic cross-clamp and cardiopulmonary bypass duration, decreased operative and ventilation time, and shorter intensive care unit and total hospital stay (Santarpino, Pfeiffer, Concistré et al. 2013; Meco, Miceli, Montisci et al. 2018; Spadaccio, Alkhamees, and Al-Attar, 2019). These variables are all well-documented determinants of morbidity and mortality in AVR. Sutureless aortic valve replacement is typically done via median sternotomy but is also amenable via less invasive options such as mini sternotomy and right anterior thoracotomy (Miceli, Murzi, Gilmanov et al. 2014). These minimally invasive options have shown to reduce bleeding, blood transfusions, incidence of atrial fibrillation, post-operative infections, and ventilation times (Brown, McKellar, Sundt et al. 2009; Gilmanov, Bevilacqua, Murzi et al. 2013). In any case, the interventional burden on the patient is drastically reduced in SU-AVR compared to SAVR.

Currently, three different sutureless bioprostheses are approved for clinical use: the Enable (Medtronic Inc.), Intuity (Edwards Lifesciences Corp.) and the Perceval (Sorin Biomedica Cardio Srl) sutureless valves (Spadaccio, Alkhamees, and Al-Attar, 2019). Indications for SU-AVR are equal to those for SAVR. This technology is especially useful for patients with multiple comorbidities or patients requiring multiple cardiac surgery procedures. This was highlighted in one study that showed that SU-AVR was associated with better hemodynamic outcomes in high-risk elderly patients who underwent multiple cardiac procedures versus SAVR (Hanedan, Ali Yuruk, Ihsan Parlar et al. 2018). Sutureless valves have been shown to reduce aortic cross-clamp and cardiopulmonary bypass times along with decreased duration of the surgical procedure in comparison with traditional surgical aortic valve replacement. This is significant, as increased aortic cross clamp time is an independent predictor of severe cardiovascular morbidity (Ranucci, Frigiola, Menicanti et al. 2012). For every 1-minute increase in cross clamp time, there is a 1.4% increased risk of stroke, acute kidney injury, impaired ejection fraction and periprocedural mortality. Better early mortality in SU-AVR versus SAVR may be attributed to the time saving nature of the procedure through shorter aortic cross clamp and cardiopulmonary bypass times. Sutureless valves are not only recommended for high-risk patients with comorbidities. They are also recommended as first line treatment for patients with anatomical complications such as a small aortic annulus, delicate aortic wall, or porcelain aorta. Moreover, it is indicated for patients requiring a redo operation, or patients requiring a concomitant cardiac surgical procedure (Gersak, Fischlein, Folliguet et al. 2016). One of the main drawbacks of SU-AVR is the risk for paravalvular leak and the need for pacemaker implantation. Reported incidences of pacemaker implantation following SU-AVR ranges from 5.6% to 9.1% which is worse than SAVR (3%) (Hurley, O'Sullivan, Segurado et al. 2015; Chandola, Teoh, Elhenawy et al. 2015). Major complications of SU-AVR include transient ischemic attack, stroke, myocardial infarction, kidney failure and infection of the surgical site (Ensminger, Fujita, Bauer et al. 2018).

Transcatheter Aortic Valve Implantation: Indications, Technique, and Outcomes

Transcatheter aortic valve implantation was first implemented in humans in 2002 and since then, has evolved as a minimally invasive option for AVR (Cribier, Eltchaninoff, Bash et al. 2002). It was originally designed for high-risk patients with severe aortic stenosis who were unfit for cardiac surgery. Recently, however, TAVI has been trialed in low to intermediate risk patients with aortic stenosis and results are encouraging. The most common approach for TAVI is the transfemoral approach where a catheter is inserted through the femoral artery and advanced to the diseased aortic valve (Oliemy and Al-Attar. 2014). Once at the aortic annulus, deployment of the valve is accomplished by a balloon-expandable (Edwards SAPIEN valve), or self-expandable valve

(Medtronic Evolut R valve). Currently, only two TAVI valves are FDA-approved: the balloon-expandable SAPIEN valve (Edwards Lifesciences) and the self-expandable CORE valve (Medtronic) (Mahmaljy, Tawney and Young, 2017). The newest generation of Medtronic valve is the EVOLUT-R and has now entered clinical trials for evaluation.

In addition to the transfemoral approach, other methods for TAVI include the transapical and subclavian approach, but these are commonly reserved for patients with severe peripheral vascular disease and have yet to gain widespread acceptance (Oliemi and Al-Attar. 2014). The minimally invasive nature of transcatheter-based aortic valve replacement is well represented in the literature by shorter in-hospital stay and minor vascular complications (Thyregod, Steinbrüchel, Ihle et al. 2015). However, TAVI typically presents with more conduction abnormalities requiring permanent pacemaker and are limited in patients with bicuspid aortic valves (Shinn, Altarabsheh, Deo et al. 2018). There are also significant concerns about paravalvular leak, as PVL is more common in TAVI compared to SAVR and SU-AVR. Nevertheless, TAVI was meant to be an effective alternative to conventional surgical aortic valve replacement and recent studies have now directly compared both procedures head-to-head.

Results

TAVI versus SAVR

The use of TAVI was originally intended for patients who were considered high risk for surgery. One of the largest randomized multicenter controlled trials to our knowledge, the PARTNER 1 trial led by Mack, Leon, Smith et al. (2015) evaluated 5-year outcomes of TAVI versus SAVR in high surgical risk patients with aortic stenosis. This randomized controlled trial was performed at 25 hospitals (22 in the USA, 2 in Canada and 1 in Germany) and included 348 patients assigned to TAVI and 351 assigned to SAVR. The primary end point of the trial was all-cause mortality at one year, and secondary end points included cardiovascular mortality, stroke, repeat hospital admission, acute kidney injury, vascular complications, bleeding and NYHA functional class. The 30-day mortality rates in the TAVI and SAVR groups were 3.4% and 6.5%, respectively, a significant finding. At 5-year follow up, the risk of death from any cause was 67.8% in the TAVI group versus 62.4% in the SAVR group, which was not found to be statistically significant. Likewise, the risk of cardiovascular causes of death, stroke or transient ischemic attack, myocardial infarction, endocarditis, renal failure or need for pacemaker implantation were similar in each group. Vascular complications and paravalvular leak were significantly more common in patients who underwent TAVI, but major bleeding episodes were significantly higher in the SAVR group. Hospital readmission rates were not significant between the TAVI and SAVR group, yet patients treated with TAVI via transapical approach were readmitted to hospital 8.8% more often than patients treated with transfemoral TAVI. Ultimately, this 5-year follow up period showed that all-cause mortality, cardiovascular mortality, stroke, need for hospital readmission and NYHA functional class were similar between TAVI and SAVR. These results suggests that TAVI is a reasonable alternative to SAVR for high-risk patients with severe aortic stenosis (Mack, Leon, Smith et al. 2015). In addition, an analysis of 4 randomized controlled trials comparing TAVI to SAVR concluded that surgical aortic valve replacement improved symptoms of heart failure post-op and reduced the risk for reintervention, pacemaker insertion and PVL, while TAVI reduced bleeding risk, atrial fibrillation, and had shorter recovery time (Siemieniuk, Agoritsas, Manja et al. 2016). Other studies found that TAVI was ineffective in reducing early and mid-term all-cause mortality in high-risk patients compared to SAVR, reinforcing the fact that median sternotomy AVR is truly the gold standard for patients who have multiple comorbidities and a high risk of periprocedural and post-procedural mortality (Cao, Ang, Indraratn et al. 2013; Takagi, Niwa, Mizuno et al. 2013).

To date, there is a lack of randomized controlled trials evaluating the use of TAVI in lower risk patients. The NOTION (Nordic Aortic Valve Intervention Trial) randomized controlled trial conducted by Thyregod, Steinbrüchel, Ihle et al. (2015) compared outcomes of TAVI with SAVR in patients $\geq$ 70 years old with severe aortic stenosis. In total, 274 patients were randomized to TAVI (N = 139) using self-expanding Medtronic Inc., prosthesis versus SAVR (N = 135) on cardiopulmonary bypass. In summary, there were no statistically significant differences in rates of death from any cause after surgery. However, post-procedure, TAVI patients had lower rates of major and life-threatening bleeding, cardiogenic shock, and acute kidney injury. Moreover, hospital stay was shorter in TAVI patients versus SAVR. Two TAVI patients had cardiac perforations and one SAVR patient required concomitant CABG due to a lesion of the right coronary ostium. At 30 days post-op, more TAVI patients required a permanent pacemaker (34.1% vs 1.6%) but had a lower rate of new-onset or worsening atrial fibrillation (16.9% vs 57.8%). At 1-year follow up, the rates of permanent pacemaker implantation remained higher in TAVI treated patients versus SAVR (38% vs 2.4%) whereas rates of new-onset or worsening atrial fibrillation was lower (21.2% vs 59.4%). On one-year follow up, there were no statistically significant differences in rates of death from any cause, nor did patients require reintervention on the repaired valves. Both patients undergoing TAVI and SAVR experienced significant improvements on the NYHA functional class by day 30 and maintenance on one year follow up, but improvements were greater in the SAVR group. No significant differences were found between TAVI and SAVR regarding death from any cause, stroke, and myocardial infarction. The TAVI cohort had fewer bleeding complications, incidence of cardiogenic shock, new or worsening atrial fibrillation, and number of days hospitalized. In contrast, the SAVR group fared better in terms of NYHA functional class at 1-year post-op, conduction abnormalities requiring permanent pacemaker and aortic valve regurgitation. In summary, this randomized controlled trial revealed that TAVI appears safe and effective in low-and intermediate-risk patients, although it was not found to be superior to SAVR (Thyregod, Steinbrüchel, Ihle et al. 2015).

Findings of both the PARTNER 1 and NOTION trials are supported by a meta-analysis of 17 studies and 4873 patients which showed no significant differences in early mortality between TAVI and SAVR (Takagi, Niwa and Mizuno, 2013). Recent results from the PARTNER 3 trial confirmed that the use of TAVI extends beyond the scope of intermediate to high-risk surgical candidates and offers equivalent outcomes to SAVR in low-risk patients with aortic stenosis (Braghiroli, Kapoor, Thielhelm et al. 2020; Pibarot, Slaun, Dahou et al. 2020). However, for high-risk patients, SAVR seems to provide slightly superior outcomes versus TAVI.

TAVI versus SU-AVR

To date, there are no published randomized controlled trials directly comparing TAVI to SU-AVR. Hence, it remains difficult to determine which technology is superior. However, Meco, Miceli, Montisci et al. (2018) conducted a meta-analysis to compare outcomes of patients undergoing TAVI with those undergoing aortic valve replacement with sutureless valves. Though no randomized controlled trials were identified, six comparative studies using propensity score matching met the inclusion criteria. In total, the meta-analysis identified 731 patients who underwent TAVI and 731 patients who underwent SU-AVR. Both sets of patients were calculated to be of intermediate to high-risk patients for these procedures, with no risk-differences between the TAVI and SU-AVR group. The primary end points were death from any cause, stroke, or myocardial infarction at 1 year. The analysis of these six studies showed that the incidence of postoperative stroke, moderate or severe paravalvular leak, 30-day mortality and in-hospital all-cause mortality was significantly lower in the SU-AVR group. Though patients in the SU-AVR group required more blood transfusion versus the TAVI group, there were significantly less major vascular complications with sutureless valves. Neither group had significant differences in postoperative pacemaker implantation, postoperative kidney failure and length in the intensive care unit post-op. On both one and two-year follow up, survival was significantly better in the SU-AVR group with a 65% and 62% risk reduction in mortality, respectively. Moreover, there was a 50% risk reduction in early all causes of death in the SU-AVR group. Although the power of this meta-analysis is limited due to a relatively low number of patients and absence of randomized controlled trials, it ultimately revealed that SU-AVR is associated with better early and mid-term outcomes versus TAVI in intermediate-to high-risk patients. Sutureless aortic valve replacement could improve outcomes for patients who are still considered in the grey zone of risk, and who might benefit from a surgical approach instead of TAVI. Interestingly, several studies have highlighted the advantages of sutureless valve technology in intermediate and high-risk patients (Glauber, Ferrarini and Miceli, 2015), which suggests that this minimally invasive approach to aortic valve replacement may become a real alternative to the TAVI procedure in the future.

It is worth noting that TAVI is a validated and an effective alternative in patients with a high surgical risk, as demonstrated by Mack, Leon, Smith et al. (2015) in the PARTNER 1 trial. However, higher risk of postoperative complications such as stroke, vascular complications, need for pacemaker implantation and moderate to severe post-procedural aortic regurgitation was observed in TAVI versus patients who underwent SU-AVR.

Another recent systematic review and meta-analysis led by Shinn, Altarabsheh, Deo et al. (2018) compared the clinical outcomes between TAVI and SU-AVR. In total 621 patients underwent TAVI and 617 underwent SU-AVR. The primary end point of this study was 30-day mortality, while secondary end points were stroke, major bleeding, need for pacemaker insertion and paravalvular leak. Seven observational comparative studies were included in the meta-analysis. In the TAVI cohorts, the Sapien (Edwards Lifesciences Inc.) and CoreValve (Medtronic) were used through transapical or transfemoral approach. In the SU-AVR group, the Perceval valve (Sorin Biomedica Cardio Srl) and the Enable valve were used and administered via right anterior minithoracotomy or median sternotomy. The analysis revealed that 30-day mortality was significantly lower in the SU-AVR group versus patients who received TAVI. Postprocedural stroke rates were lower in the SU-AVR group (1.1%) versus TAVI (1.7%) though this was not found to be statistically significant. Moreover, incidence of significant paravalvular leak was statistically lower in patients who underwent SU-AVR (1.5%) versus TAVI (11%). Interestingly, the need for pacemaker implantation in this meta-analysis was comparable between both cohorts, a contrast from the studies led by Siemieniuk, Agoritsas, Manja et al. (2016) and Thyregod, Steinbrüchel, Ihle et al. (2015). Nevertheless, recent data supports the increased need for pacemaker implantation following TAVI (van Gils, Tchetche, Lhermusier et al. 2017). It is suggested that reason behind increased pacemaker implantation post-TAVI is related to the self-expandable nature of the CoreValve, resulting in a compression of the atrioventricular conduction system of the heart. However, a balloon-expandable valve such as the Sapien does not expand when deployed. Therefore, it has little effect on damaging or interfering with the membranous septum or the conduction system of the heart (D'Onofrio, Salizzoni, Rubino et al. 2016).

Another meta-analysis of comparative studies led by Takagi, Umemoto, and the ALICE Group (2016) aimed to determine whether SU-AVR or TAVI leads to greater clinical outcomes for patients with aortic stenosis. In total, 7 observational comparative studies were included in the analysis, with a total of 945 patients assigned to SU-AVR or TAVI. It was demonstrated that SU-AVR resulted in statistically significant reductions in mortality and paravalvular leak versus TAVI. There were no statistically significant differences in bleeding complications, acute kidney injury, and conduction abnormalities.

D'Onofrio, Salizzoni, Rubino et al. (2016) also aimed to compare early outcomes of patients undergoing TAVI and SU-AVR. In total, 2177 patients from the Italian Transcatheter Balloon-Expandable TAVI registry (ITER) were used included in the multicenter analysis. Patients received the balloon expandable Sapien and Sapien XT bioprostheses via transfemoral or transapical route. Patients who underwent SU-AVR received the Perceval bioprosthesis. It is important to note that the ratio of patients who underwent TAVI to patients who underwent SU-AVR was not equal (1885 vs 292, respectively) and both cohorts had significantly different preoperative characteristics. Nevertheless, after matching all patients, results showed patients treated with TAVI had a significantly lower rate of device success (88.8% vs 98.6%) and need for pacemaker implantation (2.8% vs 9.4%). Moreover, patients who underwent TAVI had shorter in-hospital and postoperative intensive care unit stays. Both severe and mild to moderate paravalvular leak was significantly higher in patients who underwent TAVI compared to SU-AVR. There were no statistically significant differences in 30-day mortality, 1-year mortality, stroke incidence, bleeding, or myocardial infarction. This analysis showed that both TAVI and SU-AVR provide good results in patients with severe aortic valve stenosis. Patients should ultimately receive the treatment that is best suited for their clinical characteristics and anatomy.

Another interesting point to consider is the procedural costs between TAVI and SU-AVR. One study found that although the cost of both devices is similar, the sutureless approach resulted in a cost savings of roughly $13,000 US dollars per procedure (Santarpino, Pfeiffer, Jessl et al. 2015). Importantly, when considering costs of procedure, additional risk associated with the need for reintervention must be considered. For example, paravalvular leak may lead to increased need for reintervention in patients undergoing TAVI, making the procedure even more expensive. It is noteworthy that data on cost comparison between TAVI and SU-AVR are very limited.

Discussion

Following the results of the PARTNER-3 trial, the FDA further expanded the use of TAVI valves to include patients who are low-risk for surgery, making it available for a greater patient population than originally intended (Braghiroli, Kapoor, Thielhelm et al. 2020; Pibarot, Slaun, Dahou et al. 2020). In addition, TAVI offers some benefits regarding early survival and functional status but has inferior results compared with SU-AVR. Paravalvular leak and high rates of pacemaker insertion are also ongoing concerns for TAVI as any degree of PVL leads to poor long-term survival (Mack, Leon, Smith. 2015; Santarpino, Pfeiffer, Jessl et al. 2015). Paravalvular leak is considered a significant adverse prognostic indicator of short and long-term survival, as even mild PVL is associated with increased long-term mortality. A large meta-analysis of 45 studies with 12,926 patients concluded that the presence of mild, moderate, and severe PVL post-TAVI increased 30-day mortality, 1 year mortality and overall mortality rates (Athappan, Patvardhan, Tuzcu et al. 2013). However, new generations of TAVI valves are currently being studied and device improvements have been promising. It has been reported that the third generation Sapien-3 valve significantly reduces PVL versus its second-generation Sapien-XT (Nijhoff, Abawi, Agostoni et al. 2015). Nevertheless, SU-AVR offers shorter cardiopulmonary bypass time, allows for complete excision of the diseased aortic valve, and demonstrates reduced early mortality and long-term mortality versus TAVI.

The field of aortic valve replacement is rapidly evolving in the field of cardiac surgery. Although surgical aortic valve replacement is still considered the gold standard for patients with severe aortic stenosis, less invasive techniques such as transcatheter aortic valve implantation and sutureless aortic valve replacement have emerged as safe and effective measures for many different patient populations in various categories of risk. Transcatheter aortic valve replacement has now been executed in thousands of patients in the US, Canada, and Europe with a procedural success rate of 85% to 90%. Though SU-AVR is still a relatively new technology, results from recent studies are encouraging and it may soon become part of the standard of care for AVR in cardiac surgery.

In summary, both TAVI and SU-AVR are good alternatives for high-risk patients with severe aortic valve stenosis, but SU-AVR seems to be slightly safer and more effective. However, transcatheter aortic valve implantation and sutureless aortic valve replacement are not entirely comparable procedures as their indications can be quite different from one another. Both have their advantages and drawbacks, and the decision to undergo one option over the other is likely to be individualized to the patient. Patients who are treated with TAVI experience more postoperative paravalvular leak, experience higher mortality rates and demonstrate less device success compared to SU-AVR. Some studies also suggest that TAVI has a higher risk of pacemaker implantation post-procedure and impose higher costs on the medical system than SU-AVR. As advancements are made in TAVI, it is a reasonable expectation that newer generation devices should lead to better long-term outcomes in terms of PVL and vascular complications. On the other hand, patients treated with SU-AVR experience longer postoperative length of stay in hospital, and some studies suggest a higher pacemaker implantation rate, though some studies are conflicting. Moreover, SU-AVR can be used in all patients with aortic stenosis, bicuspid or not (Shinn, Altarabsheh, Deo et al. 2018).

Currently, SAVR remains the standard of care in patients with severe aortic valve stenosis and in patients with concomitant endocarditis, congenital heart abnormalities, bicuspid aortic valve, and patients requiring redo surgery.

It is unlikely that SAVR will ever be replaced as an option for aortic valve replacement. Rather, minimally invasive procedures will provide more options for patients with severe aortic stenosis and will particularly be helpful in selected cases such as calcified aortic roots, porcelain aorta or a redo situation with patent grafts. To select the optimal method for aortic valve replacement, several factors should be considered carefully. Namely, the current state of health of the patient, the preoperative risk, the rate of device success, the risk and severity of PVL, minor and major complications, postoperative length of stay and long-term mortality. Careful consideration of these variables should position the health care team to provide the patient with the best possible chance of recovering from the AVR. For patients who are considered in the "grey zone" of risk, the search for the ideal method of valve replacement is ongoing. Future studies with longer follow-up periods are warranted to determine superiority and standard of care for selecting either transcatheter aortic valve implantation or sutureless aortic valve replacement for patients with severe aortic stenosis. We are hopeful that with time, increased experience with both TAVI and SU-AVR will provide clear guidelines in selecting the optimal technology for patients in the years to come.

References

Athappan, Ganesh, Eshan Patvardhan, E. Murat Tuzcu, Lars Georg Svensson, Pedro A. Lemos, Chiara Fraccaro, Giuseppe Tarantini et al. "Incidence, predictors, and outcomes of aortic regurgitation after transcatheter aortic valve replacement: meta-analysis and systematic review of literature." *Journal of the American College of Cardiology* 61, no. 15 (2013): 1585-1595.

Braghiroli, Joao, Kunal Kapoor, Torin P. Thielhelm, Tanira Ferreira, and Mauricio G. Cohen. "Transcatheter aortic valve replacement in low risk patients: a review of PARTNER 3 and Evolut low risk trials." *Cardiovascular diagnosis and therapy* 10, no. 1 (2020): 59.

Brown, James M., Sean M. O'Brien, Changfu Wu, Jo Ann H. Sikora, Bartley P. Griffith, and James S. Gammie. "Isolated aortic valve replacement in North America comprising 108,687 patients in 10 years: changes in risks, valve types, and outcomes in the Society of Thoracic Surgeons National Database." *The Journal of thoracic and cardiovascular surgery* 137, no. 1 (2009): 82-90.

Brown, Morgan L., Stephen H. McKellar, Thoralf M. Sundt, and Hartzell V. Schaff. "Ministernotomy versus conventional sternotomy for aortic valve replacement: a systematic review and meta-analysis." *The Journal of thoracic and cardiovascular surgery* 137, no. 3 (2009): 670-679.

Cao, Christopher, Su C. Ang, Praveen Indraratna, Con Manganas, Paul Bannon, Deborah Black, David Tian, and Tristan D. Yan. "Systematic review and meta-analysis of transcatheter aortic valve implantation versus surgical aortic valve replacement for severe aortic stenosis." *Annals of cardiothoracic surgery* 2, no. 1 (2013): 10.

Chandola, Rahul, Kevin Teoh, Abdelsalam Elhenawy, and George Christakis. "Perceval sutureless valve–are sutureless valves here?." *Current cardiology reviews* 11, no. 3 (2015): 220-228.

Cribier, Alain, Helene Eltchaninoff, Assaf Bash, Nicolas Borenstein, Christophe Tron, Fabrice Bauer, Genevieve Derumeaux, Frederic Anselme, François Laborde, and Martin B. Leon. "Percutaneous transcatheter implantation of an aortic valve prosthesis for calcific aortic stenosis: first human case description." *Circulation* 106, no. 24 (2002): 3006-3008.

D'Onofrio, Augusto, Stefano Salizzoni, Antonino S. Rubino, Laura Besola, Claudia Filippini, Ottavio Alfieri, Antonio Colombo et al. "The rise of new technologies for aortic valve stenosis: a comparison of sutureless and transcatheter aortic valve implantation." *The Journal of thoracic and cardiovascular surgery* 152, no. 1 (2016): 99-109.

Ensminger, Stephan, Buntaro Fujita, Timm Bauer, Helge Möllmann, Andreas Beckmann, Raffi Bekeredjian, Sabine Bleiziffer et al. "Rapid deployment versus conventional bioprosthetic valve replacement for aortic stenosis." *Journal of the American College of Cardiology* 71, no. 13 (2018): 1417-1428.

Fischlein, Theodor, Steffen Pfeiffer, Francesco Pollari, Joachim Sirch, Ferdinand Vogt, and Giuseppe Santarpino. "Sutureless valve implantation via mini J-sternotomy: a single center experience with 2 years mean follow-up." *The Thoracic and cardiovascular surgeon* 63, no. 06 (2015): 467-471.

Gersak, Borut, Theodor Fischlein, Thierry A. Folliguet, Bart Meuris, Kevin HT Teoh, Simon C. Moten, Marco Solinas et al. "Sutureless, rapid deployment valves and stented bioprosthesis in aortic valve replacement: recommendations of an International Expert Consensus Panel." *European Journal of Cardio-Thoracic Surgery* 49, no. 3 (2016): 709-718.

Gilmanov, Daniyar, Stefano Bevilacqua, Michele Murzi, Alfredo G. Cerillo, Tommaso Gasbarri, Enkel Kallushi, Antonio Miceli, and Mattia Glauber. "Minimally invasive and conventional aortic valve replacement: a propensity score analysis." *The Annals of thoracic surgery* 96, no. 3 (2013): 837-843.

Glauber, Mattia, Matteo Ferrarini, and Antonio Miceli. "Minimally invasive aortic valve surgery: state of the art and future directions." *Annals of cardiothoracic surgery* 4, no. 1 (2015): 26.

Hanedan, Muhammet Onur, Mehmet Ali Yuruk, Ali Ihsan Parlar, Ugur Ziyrek, Ali Kemal Arslan, Ufuk Sayar, and Ilker Mataraci. "Sutureless versus conventional aortic valve replacement: outcomes in 70 high-risk patients undergoing concomitant cardiac procedures." *Texas Heart Institute Journal* 45, no. 1 (2018): 11.

Hurley, Eoghan T., Katie E. O'Sullivan, Ricardo Segurado, and John P. Hurley. "A meta-analysis examining differences in short-term outcomes between sutureless and conventional aortic valve prostheses." *Innovations* 10, no. 6 (2015): 375-382.

Kapadia, Samir R., Martin B. Leon, Raj R. Makkar, E. Murat Tuzcu, Lars G. Svensson, Susheel Kodali, John G. Webb et al. "5-year outcomes of transcatheter aortic valve replacement compared with standard treatment for patients with inoperable aortic stenosis (PARTNER 1): a randomised controlled trial." *The Lancet* 385, no. 9986 (2015): 2485-2491.

Leon, Martin B., Craig R. Smith, Michael J. Mack, Raj R. Makkar, Lars G. Svensson, Susheel K. Kodali, Vinod H. Thourani et al. "Transcatheter or surgical aortic-valve replacement in intermediate-risk patients." *New England Journal of Medicine* 374, no. 17 (2016): 1609-1620.

Mack, Michael J., Martin B. Leon, Craig R. Smith, D. Craig Miller, Jeffrey W. Moses, E. Murat Tuzcu, John G. Webb et al. "5-year outcomes of transcatheter aortic valve replacement or surgical aortic valve replacement for high surgical risk patients with aortic stenosis (PARTNER 1): a randomised controlled trial." *The Lancet* 385, no. 9986 (2015): 2477-2484.

Mahmaljy, Hadi, Adam Tawney, and Michael Young. *Transcatheter aortic valve replacement.* (2017).

Meco, Massimo, Antonio Miceli, Andrea Montisci, Francesco Donatelli, Silvia Cirri, Matteo Ferrarini, Antonio Lio, and Mattia Glauber. "Sutureless aortic valve replacement versus transcatheter aortic valve implantation: a meta-analysis of comparative matched studies using propensity score matching." *Interactive cardiovascular and thoracic surgery* 26, no. 2 (2018): 202-209.

Miceli, Antonio, Michele Murzi, Danyiar Gilmanov, Raffaele Fugà, Matteo Ferrarini, Marco Solinas, and Mattia Glauber. "Minimally invasive aortic valve replacement using right minithoracotomy is associated with better outcomes than ministernotomy." *The Journal of thoracic and cardiovascular surgery* 148, no. 1 (2014): 133-137.

Nijhoff, Freek, Masieh Abawi, Pierfrancesco Agostoni, Faiz Z. Ramjankhan, Pieter A. Doevendans, and Pieter R. Stella. "Transcatheter aortic valve implantation with the new balloon-expandable Sapien 3 versus Sapien XT Valve System: A propensity score–matched single-center comparison." *Circulation: Cardiovascular Interventions* 8, no. 6 (2015): e002408.

Nishimura, Rick A., Catherine M. Otto, Robert O. Bonow, Blase A. Carabello, John P. Erwin, Lee A. Fleisher, Hani Jneid et al. "2017 AHA/ACC focused update of the 2014 AHA/ACC guideline for the management of patients with valvular heart disease: a report of the American College of Cardiology/American Heart Association Task Force on Clinical Practice Guidelines." *Journal of the American College of Cardiology* 70, no. 2 (2017): 252-289.

Oliemy, Ahmed, and Nawwar Al-Attar. "Transcatheter aortic valve implantation." *F1000prime reports* 6 (2014).

Pibarot, Philippe, Erwan Salaun, Abdellaziz Dahou, Eleonora Avenatti, Ezequiel Guzzetti, Mohamed-Salah Annabi, Oumhani Toubal et al. "Echocardiographic results of transcatheter versus surgical aortic valve replacement in low-risk patients: the PARTNER 3 trial." *Circulation* 141, no. 19 (2020): 1527-1537.

Ranucci, Marco, Alessandro Frigiola, Lorenzo Menicanti, Serenella Castelvecchio, Carlo De Vincentiis, and Valeria Pistuddi. "Aortic cross-clamp time, new prostheses, and outcome in aortic valve replacement." *The Journal of heart valve disease* 21, no. 6 (2012): 732-739.

Santarpino, Giuseppe, Steffen Pfeiffer, Giovanni Concistré, Irena Grossmann, Martin Hinzmann, and Theodor Fischlein. "The Perceval S aortic valve has the potential of shortening surgical time: does it also result in improved outcome?." *The Annals of thoracic surgery* 96, no. 1 (2013): 77-82.

Santarpino, Giuseppe, Steffen Pfeiffer, Jürgen Jessl, Angelo Dell'Aquila, Ferdinand Vogt, Che von Wardenburg, Johannes Schwab, Joachim Sirch, Matthias Pauschinger, and Theodor Fischlein. "Clinical outcome and cost analysis of sutureless versus transcatheter aortic valve implantation with propensity score matching analysis." *The American journal of cardiology* 116, no. 11 (2015): 1737-1743.

Shinn, Sung Ho, Salah E. Altarabsheh, Salil V. Deo, Joseph H. Sabik, Alan H. Markowitz, and Soon J. Park. "A systemic review and meta-analysis of sutureless aortic valve replacement versus transcatheter aortic valve implantation." *The Annals of thoracic surgery* 106, no. 3 (2018): 924-929.

Siemieniuk, Reed A., Thomas Agoritsas, Veena Manja, Tahira Devji, Yaping Chang, Malgorzata M. Bala, Lehana Thabane, and Gordon H. Guyatt. "Transcatheter versus surgical aortic valve replacement in patients with severe aortic stenosis at low and intermediate risk: systematic review and meta-analysis." *BMJ* 354 (2016).

Spadaccio, Cristiano, Khalid Alkhamees, and Nawwar Al-Attar. "Recent advances in aortic valve replacement." *F1000Research* 8 (2019).

Takagi, Hisato, Masao Niwa, Yusuke Mizuno, Shin-nosuke Goto, and Takuya Umemoto. "A meta-analysis of transcatheter aortic valve implantation versus surgical aortic valve replacement." *The Annals of thoracic surgery* 96, no. 2 (2013): 513-519.

Takagi, Hisato, Takuya Umemoto, and ALICE (All-Literature Investigation of Cardiovascular Evidence) Group. "Sutureless aortic valve replacement may improve early mortality compared with transcatheter aortic valve implantation: A meta-analysis of comparative studies." *Journal of cardiology* 67, no. 6 (2016): 504-512.

Thyregod, Hans Gustav Hørsted, Daniel Andreas Steinbrüchel, Nikolaj Ihlemann, Henrik Nissen, Bo Juel Kjeldsen, Petur Petursson, Yanping Chang et al. "Transcatheter versus surgical aortic valve replacement in patients with severe aortic valve stenosis: 1-year results from the all-comers NOTION randomized clinical trial." *Journal of the American College of Cardiology* 65, no. 20 (2015): 2184-2194.

van Gils, Lennart, Didier Tchetche, Thibault Lhermusier, Masieh Abawi, Nicolas Dumonteil, Ramón Rodriguez Olivares, Javier Molina-Martin de Nicolas et al. "Transcatheter heart valve selection and permanent pacemaker implantation in patients with pre-existent right bundle branch block." *Journal of the American Heart Association* 6, no. 3 (2017): e005028.

Wilson, Ryan, Charis McNabney, Jonathan R. Weir-McCall, Stephanie Sellers, Philipp Blanke, and Jonathon A. Leipsic. "Transcatheter aortic and mitral valve replacements." *Radiologic Clinics* 57, no. 1 (2019): 165-178.

Chapter 4

Sensitivity of Various ECG Leads
to Acute and Chronic Myocardial Ischemia
in Biophysical Model

**I. A. Chaikovsky*, MD, PhD, I. O. Syropiatov
and M. M. Budnyk, PhD**
Department of Sensory Devices,
Systems and Technologies Of Contactless Diagnostics,
V. M. Glushkov Institute of Cybernetics of NAS of Ukraine,
Kyiv, Ukraine

Abstract

While ischemic heart disease related mortality rates decrease, it still remains a major cause of death in the world. One of the ways to further improve the situation and decrease the mortality rates is the development of preventive methods and strategies, including early detection of ischemia. An attempt is made in the paper to analyze the changes in electrocardiogram leads, reflecting manifestation and development of acute and chronic myocardial ischemia. These pathological changes were modelled using ECGSIM simulation program. Its straightforward approach consists of alteration of the shape of the transmembrane action potential curve in order to obtain the corresponding ECG curves. The research investigated several areas affected by ischemia and three stages of acute ischemia development and a case of chronic ischemia. In all ischemia simulation cases information obtained from precordial leads

* Corresponding Author's E-mail: illya.chaikovsky@gmail.com.

In: Horizons in World Cardiovascular Research. Volume 22
Editor: Eleanor H. Bennington
ISBN: 978-1-68507-568-2

exceeded those from limb leads and augmented limb leads. The most sensitive to simulated acute ischemia were precordial leads V3, V2, V5 and III standard lead. The differences in results obtained within the model and known clinical studies' results, are in the higher value of the V3 and V2 leads and lower value of V4 and, to some extent, V5 leads.

Keywords: ECG, simulation, leads sensitivity, acute and chronic ischemia, ECGSim, biophysical model

Introduction

Despite the fact that mortality rates from coronary heart disease are decreasing, it still remains the main cause of death in the world (World Health Organization 2020). One of the ways to further improve the situation and decrease the mortality rates is the development of preventive methods and strategies, including early detection of ischemia.

Electrocardiography (ECG) remains the most common method of noninvasive diagnosis of the cardiovascular system and cardiac pathologies, due to the low cost and the absence of contraindications for standard electrocardiography. But, unfortunately, as previous studies show (Chaikovsky et al., 2014; Baum et al., 2010) routine electrocardiography, i.e., registration of standard leads and their interpretation, does not have sufficient sensitivity and specificity to solve the problems faced by modern electrocardiography. On the other hand, as mentioned by Fainzilberg et al., (2007), there are a number of research methods that have sufficient sensitivity to detect ischemia, such as computed tomography, magnetic resonance imaging or radioisotope methods, magnetocardiography, as well as the most common and standardized method - perfusion scintigraphy of the myocardium. However, today, due to the increase in the number of people suffering from ischemic disorders, acceleration of the pace of life, and heavy workload in the healthcare system, there is an urgent need for devices that will allow patients to control their condition.

The creation of miniature portable electrocardiographic devices, which the patient uses to some extent independently, outside the doctor's office, are part of a broader trend, which is called point-of-care testing (POST), which in free interpretation means a medical test carried out directly at the patient's location, outside the doctor's office.

Apparently, the first representatives of this direction were household automatic tonometers. The mass production of household tonometers was started by OMRON in 1988, the widespread distribution of which began 20-25 years ago.

Then, 5-10 years ago, individual blood analyzers appeared, primarily glucose level analyzers. Portable electrocardiographs with a limited number of electrocardiographic leads are the 3rd wave of instruments for POST, which began at the very beginning of our century. The first such devices for mass use were apparently CheckMyHeart electrocardiographs (Great Britain).

There are currently dozens of different types of portable electrocardiographic devices on the market for individual use. Basically, these are single-channel electrocardiographs with finger electrodes. Let's list some of them, namely those that are most often mentioned in the relevant reviews: AfibAlert (USA), AliveCor/Kardia (USA), DiCare (China), ECG Check (USA), HeartCheck Pen (Canada), InstantCheck (Taiwan), MD100E (China), PC-80 (China). REKA E 100 (Singapore), Zenicor (Sweden), Omron Heart Scan (Japan), MDK (Holland).

All the listed devices have one or more international technical certificates (ISO, CE, FDA), registered as electrocardiographic devices. AliveCor/Kardia and ECG Check devices are structurally integrated with smartphones, other devices are specialized electrocardiographic consoles for mobile devices (smartphone, tablet, laptop) capable of registering an ECG signal and transmitting it over a distance without distortion. Most of the devices are available for open sale without restrictions, the manufacturers of some models (REKA E 100, ECG Check) declare that they are intended mainly for distribution by prescription. In this case, their acquisition (or temporary use) as a rule, it is covered by medical insurance. Many devices (for example, Zenicor) have a Web service that allows you to immediately bring a registered electrocardiogram in one lead to a doctor. All single-channel devices without exception have extensive and categorical disclaimers (i.e., disclaimer of liability) explaining that in case of any, even the most insignificant, symptoms of heart disease, it is necessary to consult a doctor immediately, without relying only on the results of an automatic ECG analysis in one lead.

In this regard, there is a need to create computer and mathematical models that would complement standard ECG methods to increase their informativeness and diagnostic value.

Method

Software for Heart Modelling

The standard approach to studying ischemic changes in the myocardium includes in vivo, in vitro and mathematical models that help us understand the mechanisms and causes of the disease and conduct drug testing (Glasser and Klein, 1994; Lines al., 2003). However, as Ytrhus (2006) mentions, such models lack the ability to effectively cope with a large number of mixed scenarios involving mixed factors. But the situation has changed with the development of computer technology and numerical methods that give researchers the opportunity to process large amounts of data. But still, extensive mathematical and computational training is required to work with such models.

There are several open-source projects that try to solve this problem by providing a visual programming interface: the SCIRun problem solving environment, OpenCMISS and ECGSim. Some other open-source projects that can be useful for research in the field of cardiology – Morpheus (Starruß et al., 2014), PhysioNet (Goldberger et al., 2000; Vest et al., 2018), CompuCell3D (Swat et al., 2012; Bouke et al., 2014), Chaste (Cooper et al., 2020) and CRISMON (Cardiovascular Integrated Modelling and SimulatiON) (Arthurs et al., 2021). Thus, the number of promising researchers who can contribute to the development of bioengineeringincreases.

SCIRun is a software environment for modeling, simulation and visualization of scientific problems, developed at the Center of Integrative Biomedical Computing. It is a working environment that allows users to select and connect software modules using the visual programming interface to create a workflow for bioelectric field studies (MacLeod et al., 2004), i.e., studies of brain activity (Black et al., 2021) and heart activity (Good et al, 2021; Jiang et al., 2021). The application software package for the SCIRun environment, called "ECG Forward/Inverse toolkit" is a set of modules and networks in the SCIRun system that can be used to solve forward and reverse electrocardiography problems (Burton et al., 2011). Also, this toolkit is able to exchange data and models with ECGSim and interact with Matlab.

OpenCMISS (Open Continuum Mechanics, Imaging, Signal processing and System identification) is a set of libraries and applications that provide modeling and visualization capabilities for a variety of bioengineering tasks. OpenCMISS consists of two main parts: OpenCMISS-Zinc is a cross-platform library of computing software for creating visualization and modeling applications; and OpenCMISS-Iron is a mathematical modeling environment that allows you to apply finite element analysis methods to solve various bioengineering problems. OpenCMISS aims to be not an application, but a modular, flexible library. And in its turn, as mentioned by Bradley et al., (2011), OpenCMISS uses a number of other open-source libraries for its work. It should be noted that OpenCMISS is the result of a complete reworking and modernization of the mathematical modeling environment of CMISS, work on which, in turn, began back in 1980.

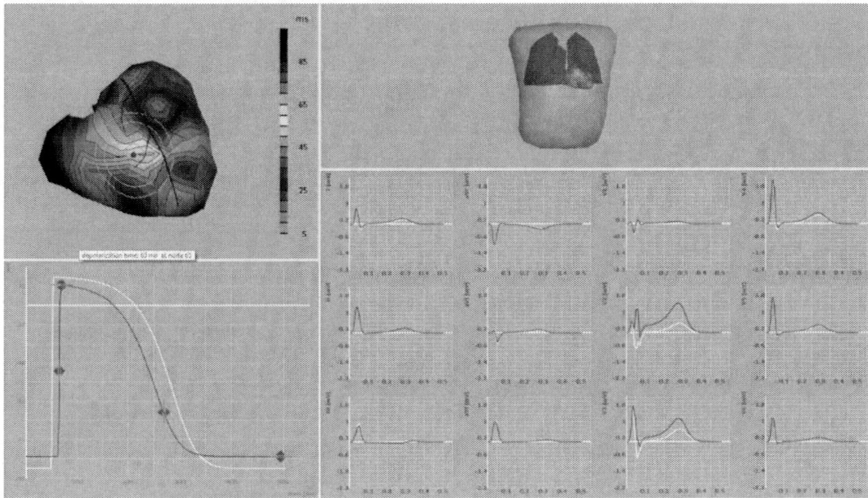

Figure 1. Example of ECGSim user interface.

ECGSIM is an interactive simulation program that allows you to study the relationship between the electrical activity of the heart and the resulting potentials on the chest: PQRST waveforms, as well as maps of the potential of the body surface. The program was developed at Radboud University Medical Center, Nijmegen, the Netherlands and is distributed under the GNU General Public License. The operation of this software is based on a mathematical model that connects an electrocardiogram with a local transmembrane potential on the surface of the myocardium (epicardium or endocardium), atria or ventricles. As introduced by van Dam, Oostendorp and van Oosterom (2010, 2011), the model uses realistic geometry of the atria, ventricles and torso, recreated using images obtained by magnetic resonance imaging. 1500 nodes are used in the model to set realistic geometry. An equivalent double layer of sources on the closed surface of the atria and ventricles (equivalent generator) is used as a source model. ECGsim allows you to change parameters describing the transmembrane potential of myocardiocytes, for example, depolarization time, repolarization time, the amplitude of the transmembrane potential in the heart or globally, the resting potential and the shape of the slope of the repolarization curve. When the input parameters are changed, the system immediately visualizes the result on the ECG (Figure 1).

Modelling Acute and Chronic Ischemia

The aim of the study was to evaluate the effect of pathological ischemic processes, created by biophysical modeling, on the electrocardiogram and to determine which ECG leads are more sensitive to such changes.

In order to select the most informative ECG leads, modeling of acute and chronic myocardial ischemia was performed using the ECGSIM modeling program. The approach consists in changing the shape of the transmembrane action potential curve and processing the corresponding obtained ECG curves. The study examined several areas affected by ischemia, three stages of acute ischemia development and a case of chronic ischemia.

In acute ischemia, there is a lack of oxygen in the myocardial cells, potassium concentrations increase and the acid-base balance changes in the direction of increasing acidity (Morena et al., 1980; Kodama et al., 1984). At the same time, the conductivity of L–calcium and sodium channels decrease and potassium channels are activated (Sato, Noma and Kurachi, 1985; Ferrero et al., 1996). This, in turn, leads to a decrease in excitability and prolonged post-polarizational refractoriness in ischemic cardiomyocytes and a reduction in the duration of their action (Shaw and Rudy, 1997; Rodriguez, Trayanova and Noble, 2006).

To simulate these changes, 15 nodes of the model were selected, 5 nodes on 3 surfaces of the heart. 5 nodes of each set are located along the heart wall from the atria to the apex. The obtained adapted ECG curves were compared with the ECG of a conditionally healthy man. The ECG curves as a whole, the qRs complex, and STT interval were considered.

Modeling of 3 stages of acute ischemia corresponding to changes occurring during 12 minutes of acute ischemia development was performed (Ferrero, Trenor and Romero, 2014; Baum, Voloshin, Popov, 2012).

In the ECGSim model, acute ischemia was modeled by reducing the repolarization time (16ms, 80ms, 131ms), reducing the amplitude of the transmembrane action potential (2mV, 3.5MV, 5mV) and reducing the resting potential (7mV, 13mV, 20mV). For example, to simulate pathological changes in the node on the anterior wall of the heart, the following parameters were used: repolarization time (281 ms, 217 ms, 167 ms), amplitude (13 mv, 11.5 mV, 10 mV) and resting potential (-78 mV, -72 mV, -65 mV). and the following values of the conditional norm in the model: 291 ms, 15 mV, -85 mV. Transmembrane action potentials of the following form were obtained (Figure 2) and an example of the ECG curves obtained at the third stage of ischemia, with the greatest changes in transmembrane potentials (Figure 3).

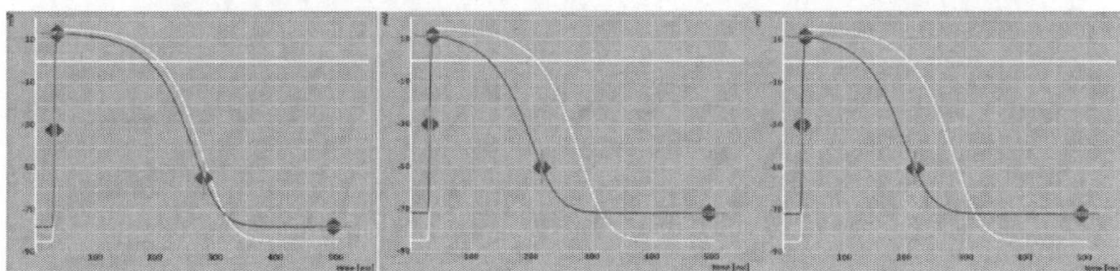

Figure 2. Transmembrane action potentials for three stages of acute ischemia development in node on the anterior surface of the heart.

The main clinical criterion for identifying acute ischemia is the dislocation (elevation or depression) of the ST segment in contiguous leads (Thygesen et al., 2018). Therefore, to begin with, we also considered the presence of significant elevation and depression of the ST segment in the simulated scenarios. For illustrative purposes, a scenario of severe acute ischemia was chosen. The results for leads on different surfaces of the heart are presented in Tables 1-3. In the tables, the values are mentioned from left to right, depending on the location of the nodes on the heart model, from the atria to the apex. Contiguous leads are the following: I, aVL, V5, V6 – the lateral surface of the heart; II, III, AVF-the lower surface of the heart, V1, V2 - the septum, V3, V4 - the front surface of the heart.

The simulation demonstrated regular changes in the dislocation of the ST segment not only in the leads "responsible" for ischemia in the corresponding zone of the left ventricular of myocardium, but also in other leads. This indicates that the scenarios of ischemia modeling used by us are adequate to the task, since they allow us to achieve changes on the electrocardiogram, which undoubtedly indicate the occurrence of ischemia.

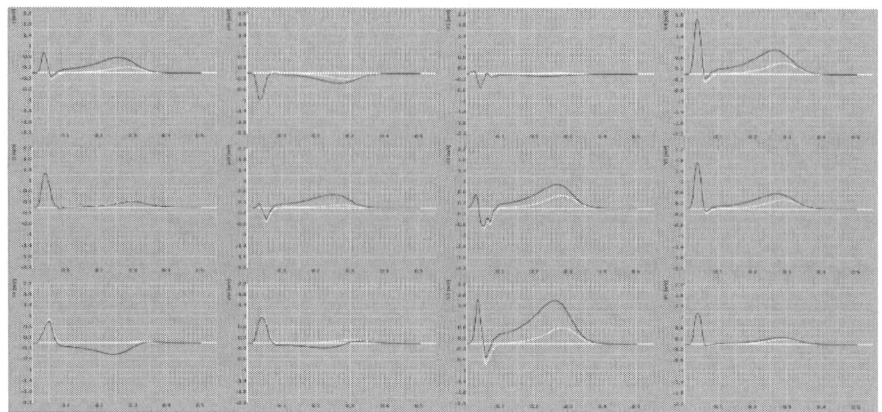

Figure 3. The ECG signals obtained for the node on the anterior surface of the heart at the third stage of acute ischemia development.

Table 1. The presence of significant elevation or depression of the ST segment in severe acute ischemia in the nodes on the anterior surface of the heart model

	Node 37	Node 12	Node 43	Node 3	Node 68
I	ST↑	ST↑	ST↑	ST↑	ST↑
II	ST↓	ST↑	ST↓	-	-
III	ST↓	ST↓	ST↓	ST↓	ST↓
aVR	-	ST↓	ST↓	ST↓	ST↓
aVL	ST↑	ST↑	ST↑	ST↑	ST↑
aVF	ST↓	ST↓	ST↓	ST↓	ST↓
V1	ST↓	ST↓	ST↓	ST↓	ST↓
V2	ST↑	ST↑	ST↑	ST↑	ST↑
V3	-	ST↑	ST↑	ST↑	ST↑
V4	ST↓	-	ST↑	ST↑	ST↑
V5	ST↓	-	ST↑	ST↑	ST↑
V6	ST↓	-	-	-	ST↑

To evaluate the obtained adapted ECG curves, we calculated the magnitude of changes as follows:

$$I = \frac{100 \times \sum |a_i - b_i|}{nP} \tag{1}$$

where ai is the value on the adapted ECG curve obtained by modeling ischemia in time i, mV; bi is the value in the ECG curve of the conditional norm in time i, mV; n is the number of counts in ECG curve, P is the peak-to-peak amplitude of the ECG signal, mV.

Table 2. The presence of significant elevation or depression of the ST segment in severe acute ischemia in the nodes on the lateral surface of the heart model

	Node 48	Node 4	Node 75	Node 20	Node 75
I	ST↑	ST↑	ST↑	ST↑	ST↑
II	-	-	ST↑	ST↑	ST↑
III	ST↓	ST↓	ST↓	-	ST↓
aVR	ST↓	ST↓	ST↓	ST↓	ST↓
aVL	ST↑	ST↑	ST↑	ST↑	ST↑
aVF	ST↑	-	-	ST↑	-
V1	ST↓	ST↓	ST↓	ST↓	ST↓
V2	ST↓	ST↓	ST↓	ST↓	ST↓
V3	ST↓	-	ST↓	ST↓	ST↑
V4	ST↓	-	ST↑	ST↑	ST↑
V5	ST↑	ST↑	ST↑	ST↑	ST↑
V6	ST↑	ST↑	ST↑	ST↑	ST↑

Table 3. The presence of significant elevation or depression of the ST segment in severe acute ischemia in the nodes on the back surface of the heart model

	Node 23	Node 90	Node 8	Node 22	Node 114
I	-	-	-	-	-
II	ST↑	ST↑	ST↑	ST↑	ST↑
III	ST↑	ST↑	ST↑	ST↑	ST↑
aVR	ST↓	ST↓	ST↓	ST↓	ST↓
aVL	-	ST↓	ST↓	ST↓	ST↓
aVF	ST↑	ST↑	ST↑	ST↑	ST↑
V1	ST↓	ST↓	ST↓	ST↓	ST↓
V2	ST↓	ST↓	ST↓	ST↓	ST↓
V3	ST↓	ST↓	ST↓	ST↓	ST↓
V4	ST↓	-	-	-	ST↑
V5	-	-	ST↑	ST↑	ST↑
V6	ST↑	ST↑	ST↑	ST↑	ST↑

As for chronic ischemia, this process, unlike acute ischemia, is characterized not by a decrease, but an increase in the refractory period (Baum,

Voloshin, Popov, 2012; Liang et al., 2019). Similar changes are characteristic of infarction and cell death (Deng et al., 2016).

Table 4. The presence of significant elevation or depression of the ST segment in chronic ischemia in the nodes on the anterior surface of the heart model

	Node 37	Node 12	Node 43	Node 3	Node 68
I	ST↑ST↓	ST↑ST↓	ST↑ST↓	ST↑ST↓	ST↑ST↓
II	ST↓ST↑	-	-	-	-
III	ST↓ ST↑	ST↓ ST↑	ST↓ ST↑	ST↓ ST↑	ST↓ ST↑
aVR	-	-	-	-	ST↓ST↑
aVL	ST↑ ST↓	ST↑ ST↓	ST↑ ST↓	ST↑ ST↓	ST↑ ST↓
aVF	ST↓ ST↑	ST↓ ST↑	ST↓ ST↑	ST↓ ST↑	ST↓ ST↑
V1	ST↓ ST↑	-	-	-	-
V2	ST↑ ST↓	ST↑ ST↓	ST↑ ST↓	ST↑ ST↓	ST↑ ST↓
V3	-	ST↑ ST↓	ST↑ ST↓	ST↑ ST↓	ST↑ ST↓
V4	-	ST↑ ST↓	ST↑ ST↓	ST↑ ST↓	ST↑ ST↓
V5	-	-	ST↑ ST↓	ST↑ ST↓	ST↑ ST↓
V6	ST↓ ST↑	-	-	-	-

Chronic myocardial ischemia was modeled as follows: the values of 3 characteristics of the transmembrane action potential changed, the deviation from the norm of each of which reflects pathological changes: a decrease in the amplitude of the action potential (by 3.5 mV to 11.5MV), a change in the resting potential from - 85 MV to -72 mV, and an increase in the duration of the horizontal phase of the plateau with the constant steepness of the curve in the repolarization phase - in the adopted model corresponds to the parameter "repolarization time" by 45ms.

Most ECG curves obtained by modeling chronic ischemia, unlike ECG curves obtained by modeling acute ischemia, are characterized by different direction of displacement of the ST segment and the T wave. While the ST segment (Point J), which connects the end of the QRS complex and the beginning of the ST segment, is shifted to one side – and the T peak is shifted to the other. The results are shown in Tables 4-6.

Although adapted curves for chronic ischemia have different character of displacement, they also show elevation and depression in corresponding contiguous leads.

Table 5. The presence of significant elevation or depression of the ST segment in chronic ischemia in the nodes on the lateral surface of the heart model

	Node 48	**Node 4**	**Node 75**	**Node 20**	**Node 75**
I	ST↑ ST↓	ST↑ ST↓	ST↑ ST↓	ST↑ ST↓	ST↑ ST↓
II	-	-	ST↑ ST↓	ST↑ ST↓	ST↑ ST↓
III	ST↓ST↑	ST↓ ST↑	ST↓ ST↑	-	ST↓ ST↑
aVR	-	ST↓ ST↑	ST↓	ST↓ ST↑	ST↓
aVL	ST↑ ST↓	ST↑ ST↓	ST↑ ST↓	-	ST↑ ST↓
aVF	-	-	-	-	-
V1	ST↓ ST↑	ST↓ ST↑	ST↓ ST↑	ST↓ ST↑	-
V2	ST↓ ST↑	ST↓ ST↑	ST↓ ST↑	ST↓ ST↑	ST↓ ST↑
V3	ST↓ ST↑	ST↓ ST↑	-	-	-
V4	-	-	-	ST↑ ST↓	ST↑ ST↓
V5	-	ST↑ ST↓	ST↑ ST↓	ST↑ ST↓	ST↑ ST↓
V6	-	ST↑ ST↓	ST↑ ST↓	ST↑ ST↓	ST↑ ST↓

Table 6. The presence of significant elevation or depression of the ST segment in chronic ischemia in the nodes on the back surface of the heart model

	Node 23	**Node 90**	**Node 8**	**Node 22**	**Node 114**
I	-	-	-	-	-
II	ST↑ ST↓	ST↑ ST↓	ST↑ ST↓	ST↑ ST↓	ST↑ ST↓
III	ST↑ ST↓	ST↑ ST↓	ST↑ ST↓	ST↑ ST↓	ST↑ ST↓
aVR	-	ST↓	ST↓	ST↓	ST↓
aVL	-	-	ST↓ ST↑	ST↓ ST↑	ST↓ ST↑
aVF	-	ST↑ ST↓	ST↑ ST↓	ST↑ ST↓	ST↑ ST↓
V1	ST↓ ST↑	ST↓ ST↑	ST↓ ST↑	ST↓ ST↑	ST↓ ST↑
V2	ST↓ ST↑	ST↓ ST↑	ST↓ ST↑	ST↓ ST↑	ST↓ ST↑
V3	ST↓ ST↑	ST↓ ST↑	ST↓ ST↑	ST↓ ST↑	ST↓ ST↑
V4	ST↓ ST↑	-	-	-	ST↑ ST↓
V5	-	-	-	ST↑ ST↓	ST↑ ST↓
V6	ST↑ ST↓	ST↑ ST↓	ST↑ ST↓	ST↑ ST↓	ST↑ ST↓

Results and Discussion

Acute Ischemia

Averaging the values obtained from nodes located on the same wall, we obtained the following results (Figures 4-6).

Most sensitive to acute ischemia modelled on frontal heart wall were precordial lead V3, V4, V2 and limb leads III, aVL, and I. As for lateral surface: precordial leads V5, V6, V2, V1 and limb leads I, aVR, aVL. Sensitive to acute ischemia modelled on the back surface of the heart were precordial leads V2, V3, V1 and limb leads II, III, and aVF.

In addition, averaging the 3 acute ischemia stages we obtained the next result (Figure 7).

In all cases of acute ischemia modeling, the information received from precordial leads exceeded that from limb leads and augmented limb leads. The most sensitive to the modeling of acute ischemia were the precordial leads V2 and V3, as well as the III standard lead.

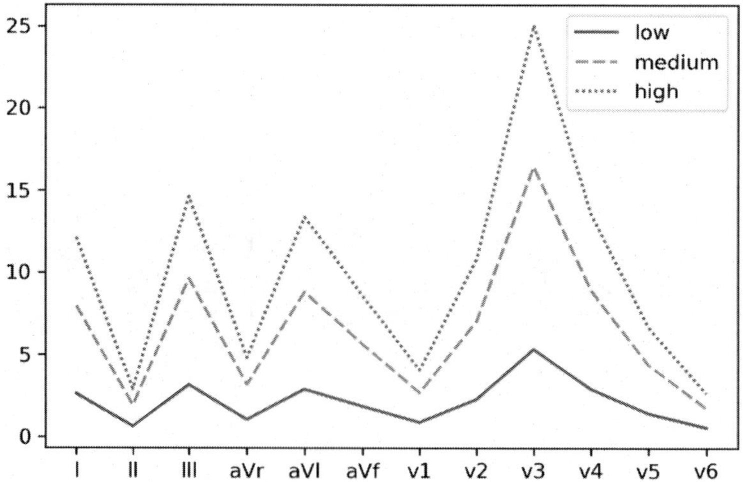

Figure 4. A graph of averaged values for nodes located on the anterior surface of the heart.

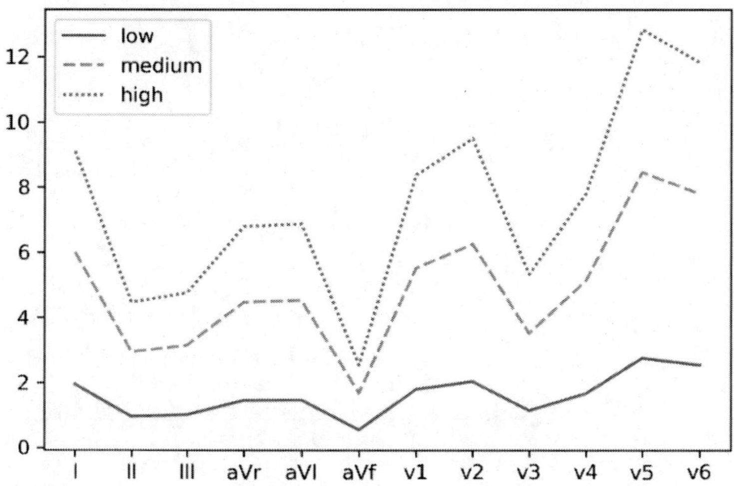

Figure 5. A graph of averaged values for nodes located on the lateral surface of the heart.

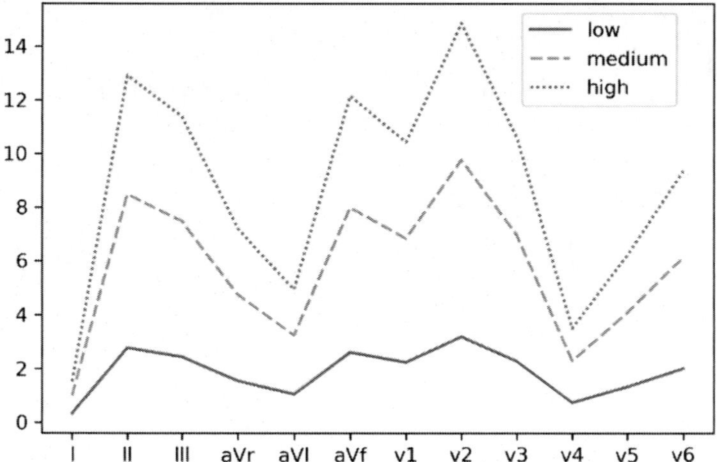

Figure 6. A graph of averaged values for nodes located on the back surface of the heart.

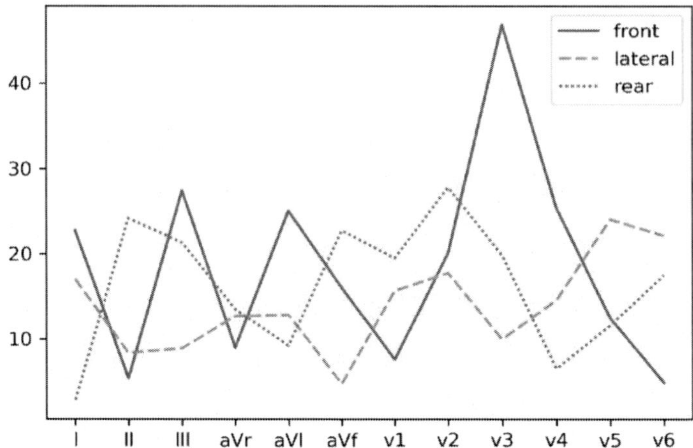

Figure 7. A graph of averaged values for different locations of the heart in acute ischemia modelling.

Chronic Ischemia

Having evaluated the results similarly to the assessment in case of acute ischemia, the following results were obtained (Figure 8).

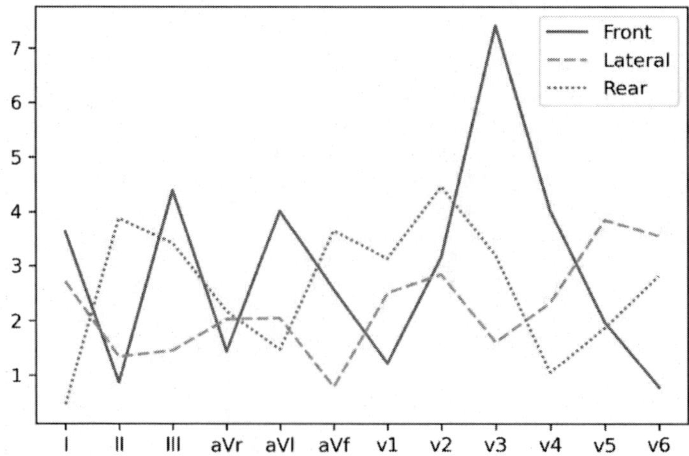

Figure 8. A graph of averaged values for different locations of the heart in chronic ischemia modelling.

It should be noted that a simulation of chronic ischemia with changes in the affected area was also performed – by increasing and decreasing the area by 15 mm and modeling a lesion passing through all layers of the heart - a transmural lesion for the affected area of the standard (within the framework of the model used) size. In general, various changes in the parameters of the affected area do not lead to drastic changes in the shape of adapted the ECG curves.

Conclusion

The results were averaged for acute and chronic ischemia. The results are presented in Figures 9, 10.

The results of our biophysical modeling generally confirm the conclusions made by clinicians regarding the sensitivity of different leads to acute ischemia. We have not found any clinical studies of patients with chronic ischemia. So, in clinical studies, and in our model, precordial leads are superior to leads from the extremities. Moreover, among the limb leads, the second lead and aVR have the least sensitivity. However, other authors point to the increased specificity of the second standard lead (London et al., 1988). According to their study, among the precordial leads, the V5 lead demonstrates the greatest sensitivity, followed by V4 and then V3 and V6, and within our model, the V3 lead showed the greatest sensitivity, followed by V2 and V5, V6.

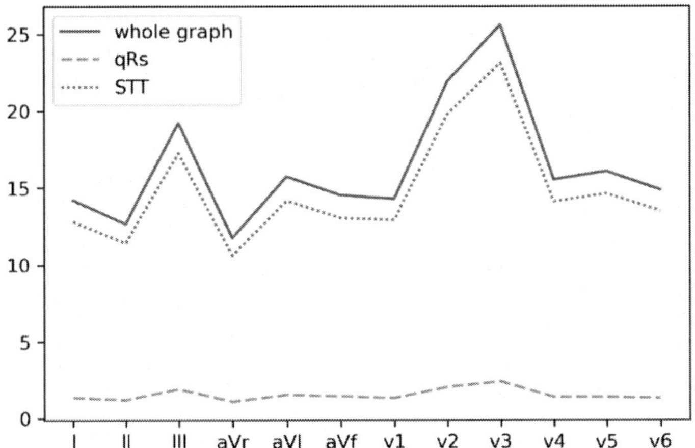

Figure 9. A graph of averaged values for acute ischemia modelling.

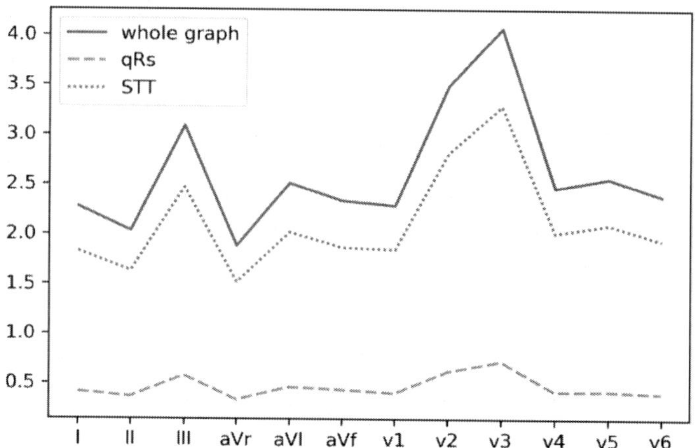

Figure 10. A graph of averaged values for acute ischemia modelling.

In its turn, among the limb leads in our model, the third standard lead from the extremities demonstrated the greatest sensitivity, followed by aVL. We explain this discrepancy by the peculiarities of the biophysical model of the electric generator of the heart, which we used(apparently).

In brief, the differences in results obtained within the model and known clinical studies' results, are in the higher value of the V3 and V2 leads and lower value of V4 and, to some extent, V5 leads.

The difference in the sensitivity of certain leads is not great between chronic and acute ischemia and consists mainly in the difference in absolute values and greater sensitivity of the STT segment in acute ischemia than in chronic. The ratio of leads in relation to their sensitivity to ischemia in both these cases is the same. However, significant differences are observed in the degree of these changes, that is, in their magnitude. In acute ischemia, these changes are significantly greater than in chronic. For qRs complex –332%, STT – 700%, for the whole graph– 625%.

As it was shown above, clinical studies investigating the sensitivity of different leads concern only patients with acute myocardial ischemia, at the same time, the number of patients with chronic ischemia is certainly greater, therefore, our modeling fills a significant gap in knowledge regarding the choice of optimal cardiac leads in such an extensive category of patients.

Conducting on other models is relevant to confirm the results obtained.

Acknowledgments

The authors want to express their sincere gratitude to Prof. Adriaan von Oosterom, Drs. Thom Oostendorp and Peter van Dam for their outstanding development of ECGSIM software.

References

Arthurs Cristopher J., Khlebnikov Rostislav, Melville Alex, Marčan Marija, Gomez Alberto, Dillon-Murphy Desmond, Cuomo Federico, et al., 2021. "CRIMSON: An open-source software framework for cardiovascular integrated modelling and simulation" *PLoS Computational Biology* 17(5):e1008881. doi:10.1371/journal.pcbi. 1008881.

Baum O. V., Chaikovsky I. A., Popov L. A., Voloshin V. I., Fainzilberg L. S., and M. M. Budnyk. 2010. "Electrocardiographic image of myocardial ischemia: Real measurements and biophysical models"*Biophysics* 55(5):812–821.

Baum O. V., Voloshin V. I., and L. A. Popov. 2012. "Electrocardiographic image of myocardial ischemia: Real measurements and biophysical models. Part II" *Biophysics* 57:668-675.

Black Shana R., Janson Andrew, Mahan Mark, Anderson Jeffrey, and Christopher R. Butson. 2021. "Identification of Deep Brain Stimulation Targets for Neuropathic Pain After Spinal Cord Injury Using Localized Increases in White Matter Fiber Cross-Section" *Neuromodulation: Technology at the Neural Interface.* doi:10. 1111/ner.13399.

Bradley Chris, Bowery Andy, Britten Randall, Budelmann Vincent, Camara Oscar, Christie Richard, Cookson Andrew, et al., 2011. "OpenCMISS: a multi-physics & multi-scale computational infrastructure for the VPH/Physiome project" *Progress in Biophysics and Molecular Biology* 107(1):32-47.doi:10.1016/j.pbiomolbio. 2011.06.015.

Burton Brett M., Tate Jess D., Erem Burak, Swenson Darell J., Wang Dafang F., Steffen Michael, Brooks Dana H., van Dam Peter M. and Rob S. Macleod. "A toolkit for forward/inverse problems in electrocardiography within the SCIRun problem solving environment" in *2011 Annual International Conference of the IEEE Engineering in Medicine and Biology Society*, 2011, pp. 267-270, doi:10.1109/IEMBS.2011.6090052.

Chaikovsky I. A., Baum O. V., Popov L. A., Voloshin V. I., Budnik N. N., Frolov Yu. A., and A. S. Kovalenko. 2014. "Parameters of cardiac muscle repolarization on electrocardiogram in case of changes of anatomical and electrical position of the heart" *Biophysics* 59(5):820–828.

CompuCell3D. 2021. *FrontPage – CompuCell3D* Accessed October 11. https://compucell3d.org.

Cooper Fergus R., Baker Ruth E., Bernabeu Miguel O., Bordas Rafel, Bowler Louise, Bueno-Orovio Alfonso, Byrne Helen M., et al., 2020. "Chaste: Cancer, Heart and Soft Tissue Environment" *The Journal of Open Source Software* 5(47): 1848. doi: 10.21105/joss.01848.

de BoerBouke A., Le GarrecJean-François, ChristoffelsVincent M., MeilhacSigolène M., and Jan M. Ruijter. 2014. "Integrating multi-scale knowledge on cardiac development into a computational model of ventricular trabeculation" *Wiley Interdisciplinary Reviews: Systems Biology and Medicine* 6(6):389-397.doi:10.1002/ wsbm.1285.

Deng Dongdong, Arevalo Hermenegild J., Prakosa Adityo,Callans David J., and Natalia A. Trayanova. 2016. "A feasibility study of arrhythmia risk prediction in patients with myocardial infarction and preserved ejection fraction" *Europace* 18(4): iv60-iv66.doi:10.1093/ europace/euw351.

ECGSIM. 2021. *"ECGSIM: The interactive ECG tool for reasearch and education"* Accessed October 12. https://www.ecgsim.org.

Fainzilberg, Leonid., Chaikovsky, Illia., Auth-Eisernitz, Sabine, Awolin, Bernard, Ivaschenko, D. and Birgit Hailer "Sensitivity and specificity of magnetocardiography, using computerized classification of current density vectors maps, in ischemic patients with normal ECG and echocardiogram" in *International Congress Series, Volume 1300*, 2007, pp. 468-471.

Ferrero Jose M., Trenor Beatriz, and Lucia Romero. 2014. "Multiscale computational analysis of the bioelectric consequences of myocardial ischaemia and infarction" *Europace* 16(3):405-415.doi:10.1093/ europace/eut405.

Github. 2021. *The Cardiovascular Integrated Modelling and Simulation Environment's Open-Source Incompressibe Navier Stokes Finite Element Flowsolver* Accessed October 16. https://github.com/carthurs/ CRIMSONFlowsolver.

Glasser R. N. A. and W. Klein. 1994. "Contractile failure in early myocardial ischemia: Models and mechanisms" *Cardiovascular Drugs and Therapy* 8(6):813–822.

Goldberger Ary L., Amaral Luis A., Glass Leon, Hausdorff Jeffrey M., Ivanov Plamen C., Mark Roger G., Mietus Joseph E., Moody George B., Peng Chung-Kang, and H. Eugene Stanley. 2000 "PhysioBank, PhysioToolkit, and PhysioNet: components of a new research resource for complex physiologic signals" *Circulation* 101(23):e215-220. doi.org/10.1161/01.CIR.101. 23.e215.

Good Wilson W., Zenger Brian, Bergquist Jake A., Rupp Lindsay C., Gillette Karli K, Gsell Matthias A. F., Plank Gernot, and Rob S. MacLeod. 2021.

"Quantifying the spatiotemporal influence of acute myocardial ischemia on volumetric conduction velocity" *Journal of Electrocardiology* 66:86-94. doi: 10.1016/j.jelectrocard.2021.03.004.

Jiang X., Font J. C., Bergquist J. A., Zenger B., Good W. W., Brooks D. H., MacLeod R. S., and L. Wang. "Deep Adaptive Electrocardiographic Imaging with Generative Forward Model for Error Reduction," in *Functional Imaging and Modeling of the Heart: 11th International Conference*, Vol. 12738, 2021, Springer Nature, pp. 471.

Kodama Itsuo, Wilde Arthur, Janse Michiel J., Durrer Dirk and Kazuo Yamada. 1984. "Combined effects of hypoxia, hyperkalemia and acidosis on membrane action potential and excitability of guinea-pig ventricular muscle" *Journal of Molecular and Cellular Cardiology.* 16(3):247-259. doi.org/10.1016/S0022-2828(84)80591-X.

Liang Cuiping, Wang Kuanquan, Li Qince and Henggui Zhang. "The Combined Effect of Myocardial Infarction and Ischemia on Excitation Wave Propagation in Ventricular Tissue" in *2019 Computing in Cardiology,* 2019, pp. 1-4.doi:10.23919/CinC49843. 2019.9005915.

Lines G. T., Buist M. L., Grottum P., Pullan A. J., Sundnes J., and A. Tveito. 2003."Mathematical models and numerical methods for the forward problem in cardiac electrophysiology"*Computing and Visualization in Science* 5(4):215–239.

London M. J., Hollenberg M., Wong M. G., Levenson L., Tubau J. F., Browner W., and D. T. Mangano. 1988. "Intraoperative myocardial ischemia: localization by continuous 12-lead electrocardiography" *Anesthesiology* 69(2):232-241.

MacLeod R. S., Weinstein O. M., de St GermainJ. Davison, Brooks D. H., Johnson C. R., and S. G. Parker. "SCIRun/BioPSE: integrated problem solving environment for bioelectric field problems and visualization" in *2004 2nd IEEE International Symposium on Biomedical Imaging: Nano to Macro* 2004, Vol. 1, pp. 640-643. doi: 10.1109/ISBI.2004.1398619.

Morena Herve, Janse Michiel J., Fiolet Jan W. T., Krieger Willem J. G., Crijns Harry and Dirk Durrer. 1984. "Comparison of the effects of regional ischemia, hypoxia, hyperkalemia, and acidosis on intracellular and extracellular potentials and metabolism in the isolated porcine heart" *Circulation Research* 46(5):634-646.

Morpheus. 2021. *Morpheus*Accessed October 14. https://morpheus. gitlab.io.

OpenCMISS. 2021. *OpenCMISS*Accessed October 12. http://open cmiss.org.

PhysioNet. 2021. *PhysioNet* Accessed October 14. https://physionet. org.

Rodriguez Blanca, Trayanova Natalia and Denis Noble. 2006. "Modeling Cardiac Ischemia" *Annals of the New York Academy of Sciences* 1080:395-414. doi:10.1196/annals.1380.029.

Sato R., Noma A., Kurachi Y., and H. Irisawa. 1985. "Effects of intracellular acidification on membrane currents in ventricular cells of the guinea pig" *Circulation Research* 57(4):553-561. doi.org/10.1161/01.RES.57.4.553.

Shaw Robin M.and Yoram Rudy. 1997. "Electrophysiologic effects of acute myocardial ischemia: a theoretical study of altered cell excitability and action potential duration" *Cardiovascular Research* 35(2):256-272. doi:10.1016/S0008-6363(97)00093-X.

Shaw Robin M. and Yoram Rudy. 1997."Electrophysiologic effects of acute myocardial ischemia. A mechanistic investigation of action potential conduction and conduction failure" *Circulation Research* 80(1):124-138. doi:10.1161/01.RES.80.1.124.

StarrußJörn, de Back Walter, Brusch Lutz, and Andreas Deutsch. 2014. "Morpheus: a user-friendly modeling environment for multiscale and multicellular systems biology" *Bioinformatics* 30(9):1331-1332.

Swat Maciej H., Thomas Gilberto L., Belmonte Julio M., Shirinifard Abbas, Hmeljak Dimitrij, and James A. Glazier. 2012. "Multi-scale modeling of tissues using CompuCell3D" in *Computational Methods in Cell Biology*, Vol. 110, edited by Anand R. Asthagiri, Adam P. Arkin, 325-366.

The NIH/NIGMSCenter for Integrative Biomedical Computing. 2021. "*SCIRun*" Accessed October 12. https://www.sci.utah.edu/cibc-software/scirun.html.

Thygesen Kristian, Alpert Joseph S., Jaffe Allan S., Chaitman Bernard R, Bax Jeroen J., White Harvey D, et al., 2018. "Fourth Universal Definition of Myocardial Infarction (2018)" *Circulation* 138(20): e618-e651. doi:10.1161/CIR.0000000000000617.

University of Oxford Department of Computer Science. 2021. *Cancer, Heart and Soft Tissue Environment* Accessed October 15. https://www.cs.ox.ac.uk/chaste.

van Dam Peter M., Oostendorp Thom F. and Adriaan van Oosterom. 2011. "Interactive simulation of the activation sequence: Replacing effect by cause" *Computers in Cardiology* 38:657-660.

van Dam Peter M., Oostendorp Thom F. and Adriaan van Oosterom. "ECGSIM: Interactive simulation of the ECG for teaching and research purposes" in *2010 Computing in Cardiology,* 2010, pp. 841-844.

Vest Adriana, Da Poian Giulia, Li Qiao, Liu Chengyu, Nemati Shamim, Shah Amit J., and Gari D. Clifford. 2018. "An Open Source Benchmarked Toolbox for Cardiovascular Waveform and Interval Analysis" *Physiological Measurement* 39(10):105004. doi.org/10. 1088/1361-6579/aae021.

World Health Organization. 2020. *The top 10 causes of death*, Last modified December, 9. https://www.who.int/news-room/fact-sheets/detail/the-top-10-causes-of-death.

Ytrehus K. 2006. "Models of myocardial ischemia," *Drug Discovery Today: Disease Models* 3(3):263–271.

Chapter 5

Cardiac Magnetic Resonance Techniques to Determine Systemic Impedance in Healthy Individuals and Cardiovascular Disease States

Sara L. Hungerford[1,3,*], PhD,
Nicole K. Bart[1,3], PhD and Audrey I. Adji[1,4], PhD
[1]Department of Cardiology, St Vincent's Hospital, Sydney Australia
[2]St Vincent's Clinical School, University of New South Wales, Sydney Australia
[3]Victor Chang Cardiac Research Institute, Sydney Australia
[4]FMHHS, Macquarie University, Sydney, Australia

Abstract

The rapid uptake of cardiovascular therapeutics and device technologies has led to a renewed interest in cardiac magnetic resonance imaging (CMR) techniques to non-invasively measure vascular impedance as an estimate of systemic load of the human circulation. Impedance, by definition, expresses the relationship between pulsatile pressure and flow in an artery. Cardiac magnetic resonance imaging can accurately assess structure and function of the great arteries, including flow velocity in the ascending aorta or main pulmonary artery. Systemic impedance can be estimated by ascending aortic flow velocity data coupled with non-invasively derived central aortic pressure data. In the case of pulmonary impedance estimation, non-invasive pressure measurement has not yet

[*] Corresponding Author's E-mail: sara.hungerford@svha.org.au.

In: Horizons in World Cardiovascular Research. Volume 22
Editor: Eleanor H. Bennington
ISBN: 978-1-68507-568-2

been demonstrated to be feasible. As such, a hybrid approach of main pulmonary artery CMR-flow velocity data and pulmonary artery pressure by invasive right heart catheterisation is described. The following Chapter reviews existing and upcoming CMR techniques to evaluate systemic and pulmonary impedance in healthy individuals and cardiovascular disease states.

Keywords: applanation tonometry, cardiac magnetic resonance imaging, pulmonary impedance, systemic impedance, valvulo-arterial impedance

Abbreviations

AA	ascending aorta;
AS	aortic valve stenosis;
AT	applanation tonometry;
CMR	cardiac magnetic resonance;
FFT	fast Fourier transformation;
LV	left ventricular;
MPA	main pulmonary artery;
PA	pulmonary artery;
Pn	derived central aortic pressure;
PH	pulmonary hypertension;
PWV	pulse wave velocity;
Qn	aortic flow velocity product;
RHC	right heart catheterisation;
RV	right ventricular;
TAVI	transcatheter aortic valve implantation;
VAL	valvulo-arterial load;
VTF	velocity transfer function;
Z_C	characteristic impedance;
Z_{IN}	input impedance;
$Z_{VA\text{-}INS}$	valvulo-arterial impedance-instantaneous.

Introduction

The past decade has seen considerable growth in therapeutics and device technologies to treat a variety of cardiovascular disease states. With these advances, clinicians have been increasingly challenged by the need to differentiate between those that will benefit from intervention and those that will not. The hemodynamic loading conditions in patients with valvular heart disease or congestive cardiac failure are often unique and not adequately accounted for using traditional echocardiography techniques. Load independent assessment of cardiac function requires simultaneous measurement of ventricular pressure and volume in order to determine the relationship between these two parameters at various points in the cardiac cycle [1]. Cardiac magnetic resonance imaging (CMR) techniques to assess function and structure of the heart and great vessels for estimating impedance of the systemic and pulmonary circulations are uniquely placed in this regard.

Cardiac magnetic resonance assessment of flow using velocity-encoded sequences is well established [2]. So too are applanation tonometry (AT) techniques to accurately and non-invasively measure central aortic pressure by a carotid or radial approach [3, 4]. Simultaneous, non-invasive measurement of ascending aortic (AA) pressure and flow has resulted in the development of several CMR methods to describe systemic impedance in healthy individuals and cardiovascular disease states. These methods are reviewed in detail below. A hybrid approach of main pulmonary artery (MPA) flow velocity data and pulmonary arterial (PA) pressure waveform from right heart catheterisation (RHC) have also been applied to derive impedance of the pulmonary circulation. The following Chapter provides an overview of key concepts, as well CMR-derived methods to measure systemic and pulmonary impedance in healthy individuals and cardiovascular disease states.

Defining Impedance of the Circulation

Vascular impedance represents properties of the whole circulation and characterises the hydraulic load of the circulation presented to the heart. When the general term 'impedance' is applied to a vascular bed, it is usually referred to "input impedance" (Z_{in}), this being the relationship between pulsatile pressure and pulsatile flow recorded in an artery feeding a particular vascular bed. Z_{in} can be estimated with the following complex equation:

$$Z_{in} = \frac{|P|}{|Q|} cos(\beta - \phi),$$

where $|Z_{in}| = |P| \div |Q|$ is the modulus and $\theta = (\beta - \phi)$ is the phase of the impedance [5, 6]. It is determined by relating corresponding frequency components of arterial pressure and flow waves acquired simultaneously in that artery site, and each of the corresponding harmonics' modulus and phase are plotted against frequency. This ratio between pulsatile pressure and flow involves input from all the vascular tree beyond that site and depends upon the local arterial properties and the properties of all vessels in the vascular bed beyond [7]. The term characteristic impedance (Z_C) on the other hand, refers the relationship between pulsatile pressure and pulsatile flow in an artery when these waves are not influenced by wave reflection [7]. Zc can be estimated by averaging Z_{IN} moduli over a frequency band, usually between 2 to 10 Hz [4, 11].

Using simultaneously (or near simultaneous) acquired pressure and flow data, estimates of impedance can be obtained using frequency or time domain analysis. For impedance estimation performed in the frequency domain, flow velocity and pressure waveforms are decomposed into their harmonics component using a fast Fourier transformation (FFT) for frequencies up to 10 Hz, as harmonics greater than 10 Hz can be regarded as noise [11]. Total peripheral arterial resistance (also known as systemic vascular resistance) is considered as the impedance modulus at 0 Hz, whilst Z_C is routinely estimated as the mean magnitude of Z_{IN} modulus between 2 and 10 Hz [7]. Although frequency domain analysis is a more common method of impedance determination, has a stronger basis in the physical sciences and more appropriately suited for clinical studies, it is more difficult to apply [8]. As such, impedance is often calculated in the time domain (based on an approach introduced by *Dujardin and Stone*) using the "up-slope method," utilising the initial upstroke of arterial pressure and flow waves during the early phase of left ventricular ejection [9]. Calculation of impedance in the time domain is based on the assumption that pressure and flow are linear and measured simultaneously at the same location [8], however this is not necessarily the case in cardiovascular disease states.

Cardiac Magnetic Resonance Methods
to Determine Systemic Impedance

Systemic impedance of the human circulation was first determined in pioneering catheter studies during the 1960's and 1970's [10-14]. It began with the introduction of steady-state analysis of arterial pulses in the frequency domain in the 1960s which showed that non-linearities in these relationships were sufficiently small to be neglected to a first approximation. However, these studies have not been actively pursued beyond the 1970s, partly because of the requirement of invasive technique and costly sensors to register arterial pressure and/or flow waveform accurately.

Systemic impedance represents properties of the whole systemic circulation and characterises the hydraulic load of systemic circulation presented to the heart. A typical Z_{IN} pattern in the ascending aorta shows a relatively high modulus at zero frequency – which is the peripheral/systemic resistance or steady-state load – then fall of modulus with increasing frequency to a minimal value around 3-4 Hz, before rising to a maximal value around twice the minimal frequency and continue to fluctuate around its Zc at higher frequencies [15, 16]. The phase (or difference in angle) value is negative at low frequencies – indicating arterial flow leading pressure – then crosses zero around the same frequency where modulus is minimum, and becomes positive at higher frequencies [15, 16]. These impedance patterns are mainly influenced by ascending aorta distensibility and arterial pulse wave velocity [4], such as with aging and cardiovascular disease.

Non-invasive characterization of systemic impedance remained challenging until the introduction of CMR over a decade later. With the introduction of non-invasive arterial pressure measurement using AT it is now possible to combine pressure data with CMR-acquired flow data to estimate vascular impedance [17]. Several studies have since validated systemic impedance estimation using combined CMR and AT methods [18-21]. These methods are reviewed below. The combination of arterial pressure and flow, as well as LV volume can allow a more comprehensive evaluation of LV function, stiffness of the elastic arteries due to aging, and interaction between the LV and the vasculature. Estimation of systemic vascular impedance independent of LV contractility is valuable in a range of clinical conditions including hypertension, heart failure, valvular heart disease and ischemic heart disease.

In 2016, Adji et al. first described an operator-independent method of calibrated aortic pressure waveform acquisition via the use of a purpose-built, free-standing arterial bracelet radial tonometer [11, 22]. This technique permitted simultaneous acquisition of aortic pressure (derived from radial tonometric pressure using a validated mathematical function), CMR flow and LV volume data in healthy human subjects for the first-time using frequency domain analysis [20]. This technique has since been replicated in healthy individuals and those with cardiovascular disease states (Figures 1 and 2) [21, 23].

Non-simultaneous measurement of central aortic pressure and CMR flow has also been described using carotid AT following CMR exam [18, 19]. In 2015, Bollache et al. reported on seven different methods for the estimation of Z_C and found that methods based on 95% of peak flow, as well as those based on derivative peaks and up-slopes could be easily integrated into a clinical workflow [18]. Carotid tonometry is less favoured in this setting, however, as it is not able to record pressure simultaneously with CMR flow, artifact is common, and it can activate baroreceptors so as leading to reflex changes in heart rate and arterial pressure [24].

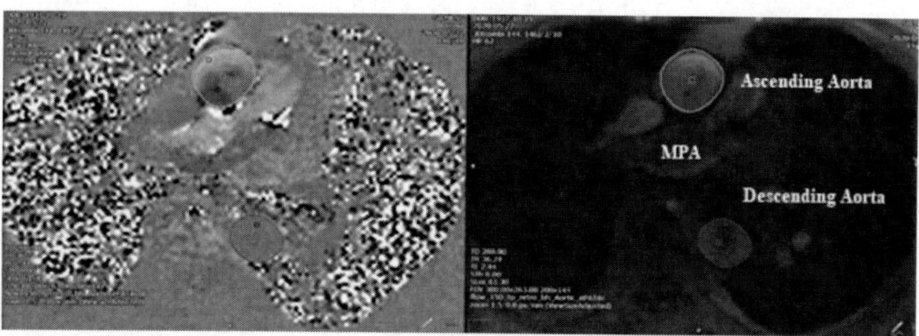

(Left) Quantitative flow velocity mapping of ascending/descending aorta at the level of the MPA.

(Right) Single cine of ascending/descending aorta at the level of the MPA and preparation for quantitative flow velocity mapping.

Abbreviations: MPA, main pulmonary artery.

Figure 1. Representative cardiac magnetic resonance aortic quantitative flow analysis.

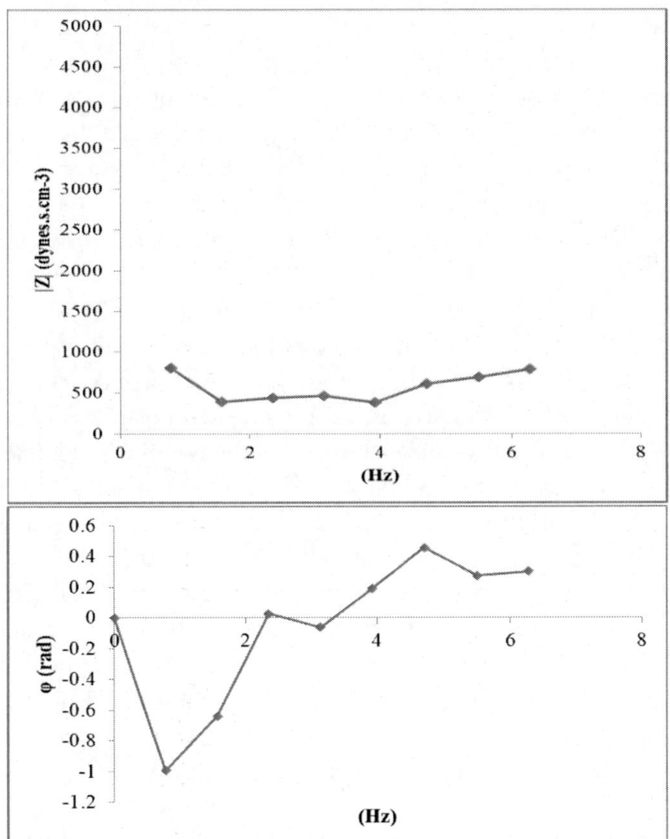

Simultaneous CMR/AT derived representative vascular load plot in a healthy young patient. Impedance phase shows crossing from zero to positive around 2Hz. Abbreviations: AT, arterial tonometry; CMR, cardiac magnetic resonance.

Figure 2. Representative vascular load plot in healthy young patient.

Cardiac Magnetic Resonance Methods to Determine Pulmonary Impedance

Impedance of the pulmonary arterial system was first described in invasive studies during the 1970's and 80's [25-28]. The technical aspects of custom-designed right heart multi-sensory catheters containing solid-state pressure sensors and electromagnetic flow velocity probes have been described previously [25-28]. Difficulties including frequency response, drift characteristics and calibration techniques have limited its widespread use [28] and as such, has rarely been used outside of a research setting over the past three decades. More recently, right ventricular (RV)- pulmonary arterial (PA) coupling has been derived invasively from the ratio between end-systolic elastance (Ees) and effective arterial elastance (Ea) as a load independent parameter of intrinsic myocardial contractility. Calculation of Ea is not straight-forward, however, as it is derived by the creation of multiple different pressure-volume loops (through partial vena cava occlusion or by the Valsalva manoeuvre).

With the introduction of CMR, several parameters of PA stiffness have now been described - including PA compliance, distensibility, capacitance, elasticity, and stiffness index [29]. However, all these indices still require a combined approach of invasive measurement of intra-pulmonary pressures with RHC and non-invasive measurement of change in PA diameter or cross-sectional area within the cardiac cycle on CMR [29]. Completely non-invasive measures of PA stiffness (including comparison of PA diameter with aortic diameter and pulsatility), have not been demonstrated to be significantly different in patients with low or high pulmonary vascular resistance [30]. Similarly, pulse wave velocity (PWV) has been studied as a non-invasive measure of PA stiffness, but the main difficulty of measuring PWV in this setting is related to the change of the shape of pressure and flow waves with distance that makes it difficult to assign a single value.

In 2018, *Gupta* et al. used a velocity transfer function (VTF) method as a surrogate of invasive impedance in a prospective group of 20 patients undergoing hybrid RHC, echocardiography and CMR evaluation. In this study, the author(s) combined non-simultaneous acquisition of invasive impedance (RHC-Doppler) with VTF (CMR). However, whereas impedance is expressed as the ratio of moduli of pressure by flow in the frequency domain, VTF refers to the ratio of moduli of output velocity profile to input velocity profile in the frequency domain. Despite this limitation, VTF was demonstrated to be measured in a completely non-invasive manner and was found to offer high sensitivity and specificity for detection of increased PA stiffness [30]. Efforts are currently underway to assess pulsatile pulmonary impedance using a hybrid CMR and RHC approach. In patients with, or being investigated for PH, it is anticipated that readily available PA pressure and CMR flow velocity data can be coalesced in a similar manner as demonstrated for the systemic circulation to derive pulmonary impedance using frequency domain analysis.

Cardiac Magnetic Resonance Vascular Impedance Estimation in Healthy Human Ageing

Healthy Human Ageing

With ageing, the central elastic aorta progressively dilates, elongates, and becomes tortuous with stiffened and thickened walls [10]). Characteristic age-related changes in systemic flow velocity, pressure waveform and vascular impedance of the aorta by a CMR are now well described [6, 31].

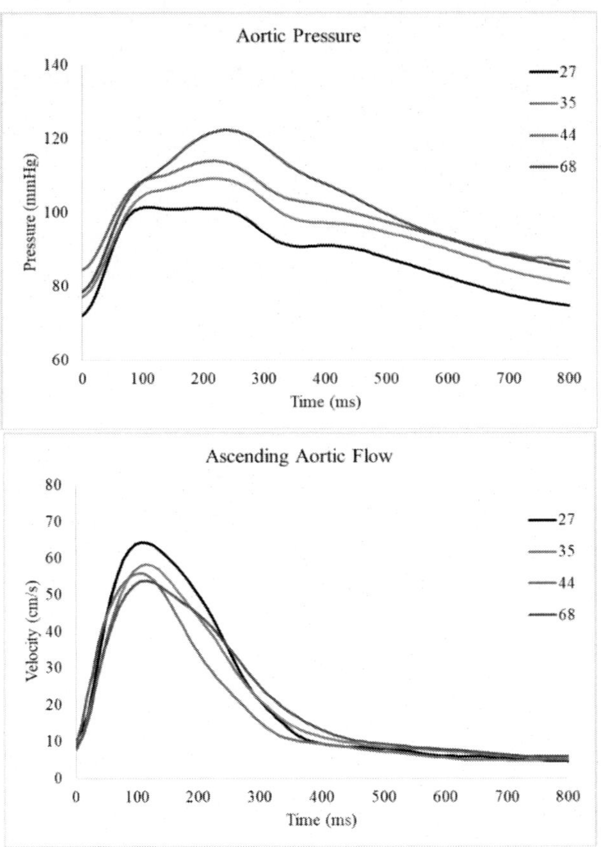

Figure 3. (Continued)

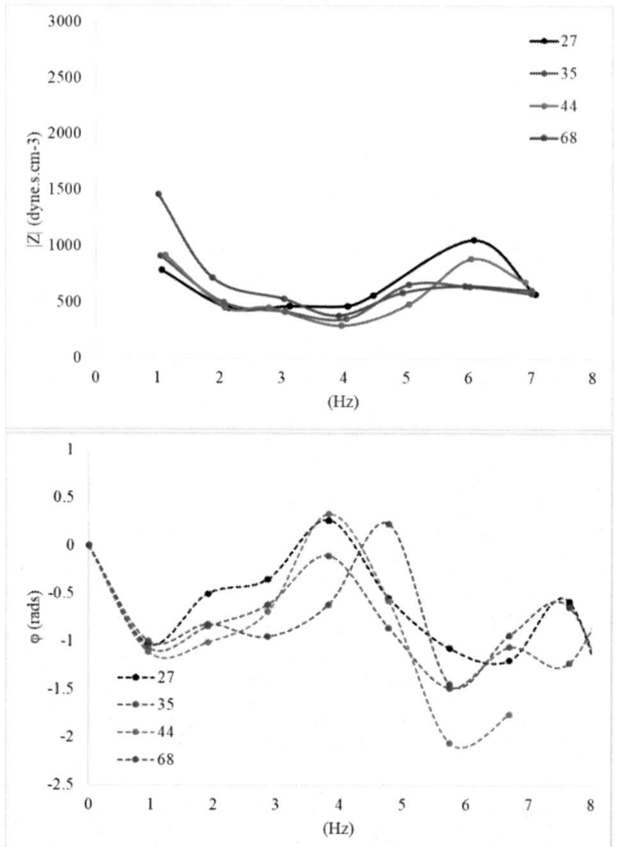

(Top) Tonometry-derived representative central aortic pressure waveform showed increased central aortic pressure with age.

(Middle) CMR-derived representative aortic flow velocity waveform showing reduced aortic flow velocity with age.

(Bottom) Simultaneous CMR/AT derived representative systemic impedance plot grouped by age. Systemic impedance phase shows similar values for the first harmonic at all ages, then increases for all age groups, crossing zero to positive values later in more elderly patients (around 3-4 Hz).

Figure 3. Representative aortic pressure, flow velocity and systemic impedance plots grouped by age.

Tonometry-derived representative central aortic pressure waveforms in healthy young patients typically show increased central aortic pressure relative to elderly patients. In one study by *Hungerford* et al., aortic unfolding was found to lead to a lower peak flow velocity in older patients [6], while *Adji* et al. described a more subtle reduction in late systolic flow [11]. Coupled with a shift in the aortic pressure waveform, stiffer older vessels were demonstrated to lead to a faster velocity of pressure pulse and earlier timing of the reflected pulse wave from the periphery, augmenting central aortic systolic pressure and yielding a greater afterload on the heart [5, 6]. Systemic vascular resistance is higher, while systemic impedance phase typically shows similar values for the first harmonic at all ages, then increases for all age groups, crossing zero to positive values later in elderly patients (around 3-4 Hz). Any alteration in systemic impedance pattern causes further mismatch between Z_C and energy expenditure of LV ejection, and an increase in pulsatile energy lost in the circulation. Additionally, mean aortic systolic pressure is increased, thus rising LV oxygen requirements and LV afterload, while mean aortic diastolic pressure is decreased, hence reducing coronary blood flow. All these changes will eventually lead to cardiac hypertrophy, decrease in cardiac output and heart failure [32]. Figure 3 shows a representative aortic pressure and flow velocity waveform and systemic impedance plots grouped by age.

Cardiac Magnetic Resonance Vascular Impedance Estimation in Cardiovascular Disease States

Aortic Valve Stenosis

In the past 5-years, two CMR methods to assess systemic impedance in patients with aortic stenosis (AS) have been described – valvulo-arterial impedance instantaneous ($Z_{VA\text{-}INS}$) and valvulo-arterial load (VAL). *Soulat* et al. [33] first described $Z_{VA\text{-}INS}$ in 2017 using CMR and non-simultaneous carotid tonometry. Valvulo-arterial impedance instantaneous is estimated by acquiring CMR velocities above the aortic valve and within the LV outflow tract, and by carotid tonometry after CMR exam. It is calculated in the time domain by combining the incident LV pulse pressure to 95% of peak flow:

$$Z_{VA\text{-}INS} = (\Delta P_{\text{-}Q95} + MaxG_{\text{-}NET}) \div \Delta Q_{\text{-}95,}$$

where $\Delta P_{\text{-}Q95}$ is the LV pressure (taken to be the same as carotid tonometric pressure) change from its end-diastolic foot to time of 95% of peak flow ($Q_{\text{-}95}$) and $MaxG_{\text{-}NET}$ is the maximum gradient calculated in the aortic valve considering pressure recovery [33]. The LV end-diastolic foot, however, occurs prior to aortic valve opening at the start of isovolumic contraction. This represents an inherent limitation of the Z_{VA-INS} index, as the LV pressure change at time of aortic valve opening is required for estimation of characteristic impedance [23].

Hungerford et al. subsequently described the VAL index in 2020. Whereas Soulat et al. [33] calculate Z_{VA-INS} as the ratio between total arterial pressure (the summation of carotid tonometric pressure as a surrogate for central aortic pressure and maximum pressure gradient of the aortic valve) and CMR ascending aortic flow, VAL is estimated as the global LV afterload. That is, VAL is derived from the simultaneous relationship between aortic pressure and flow velocity. Data obtained forms a graph of modulus and phase, plotted against frequency [23]. VAL is expressed as:

$$VAL = \frac{Pn}{Qn} e^{i(\theta n - \varphi n)},$$

where *VAL* represents global LV load, *Pn* represents derived central aortic pressure, *Qn* represents aortic flow velocity product at the MPA level, and ei(θn−φn) represents both the harmonic component of pressure and phase of impedance

VAL differs from Z_{VA-INS} as it permits (i) simultaneous acquisition of aortic pressure and flow; (ii) measures the combined LV afterload; (iii) samples the multiple flow profiles seen in patients with AS [34], and; (iv) estimates systemic impedance in the frequency domain [8]. As aortic valve stenosis and systemic hypertension represent elevated impedances in series, simple summation of these resistances (as in the case of Z_{VA-INS}) may lead to an overestimation of global LV load [23, 35]. Studies of systemic impedance estimation in patients undergoing transcatheter aortic valve implantation (TAVI) are currently underway.

Pulmonary Hypertension

Accurate quantification of pulsatile impedance of the pulmonary circulation remains challenging in patients with PH. Pulmonary hypertension is traditionally defined by elevated pulmonary artery pressures or pulmonary vascular resistance (PVR) [36]. Neither measurement, however, accounts for the pulsatile energy losses of the pulmonary circulation, and as such, neither is able to truly measure pulmonary impedance [25].

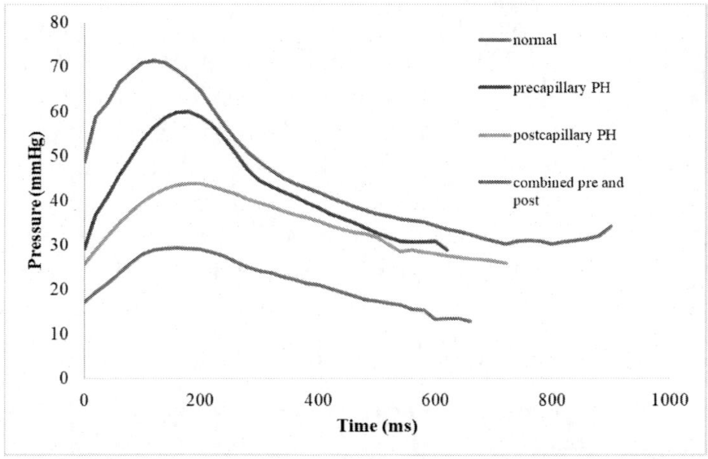

Abbreviations: PA, pulmonary artery; PH, pulmonary hypertension.

Figure 4. Representative PA pressure waveforms from different PH populations.

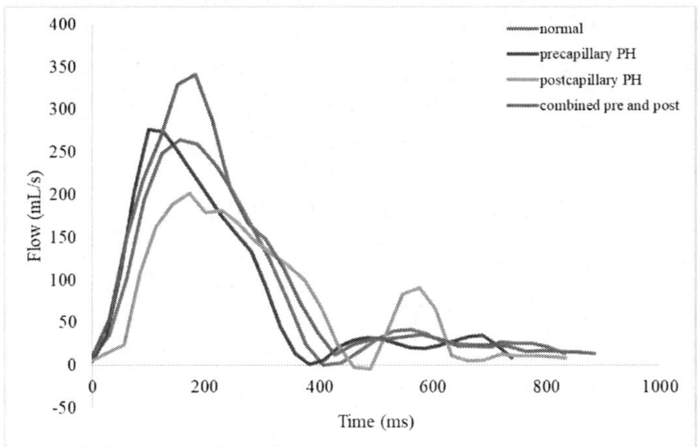

Abbreviations: CMR, cardiac magnetic resonance; PA, pulmonary artery; PH, pulmonary hypertension.

Figure 5. Representative PA CMR-derived flow velocity curves form different PH populations.

As there remains no reliable method to non-invasively measure PA pressure, CMR methods to derive pulmonary impedance have largely been confined to PH patients with dyspnoea undergoing clinically indicated RHC and CMR evaluation. Early clinical trials are underway to evaluate patients with known or suspected PH who undergo routine RHC and CMR study.

Preliminary results ahead of publication show pulmonary impedance to be reassuringly lower in patients with normal PA pressures, than those with pulmonary hypertension. Moreover, in the subset of patients with pre-capillary PH, there appears a trend towards higher pulmonary impedance values than in patients with post-capillary or mixed PH. The results of early feasibility studies are highly anticipated and validation with larger cohort studies and/or a pharmacological agent to improve RV contractility or reduce PH would be beneficial. Figure 4 shows representative PA pressure waveforms from different PH populations. Figure 5 shows representative PA CMR-derived flow velocity curves form different PH populations.

Conclusion

Difficulties in the invasive measurement of vascular impedance of the human circulation means that it is not routinely been performed. The development of enhanced CMR techniques over the past decade has provided clinicians with new methods to estimate systemic and pulmonary impedance in healthy individuals and cardiovascular disease states so as to better uncouple complex ventricular-vascular interactions. Insights gained from impedance estimation in elderly patients, those with valvular heart disease, or congestive cardiac failure, are expected to compliment conventional echocardiographic indices in the future, which at times have become antiquated and confused. It is anticipated that the ability to determine gold standard afterload in combination with gold standard contractility will promote the transition of CMR techniques for impedance determination into more routine clinical practice, where the appreciation of the interaction between ventricular function and arterial load is increasingly being sought [1, 37, 38].

Disclosures

All authors have reported that they have no relationships relevant to the contents of this paper to disclose.

Funding

All other authors have reported that they have no funding disclosures relevant to the contents of this paper to disclose.

References

[1]	Merillon JP, Ennezat PV, Guiomard A, Masquet-Gourgon C, Aumont MC, Gourgon R. Left ventricular performance is closely related to the physical properties of the arterial system: Landmark clinical investigations in the 1970s and 1980s. *Archives of cardiovascular diseases*. 2014;107(10):554-62.

[2]	Dyverfeldt P, Bissell M, Barker AJ, Bolger AF, Carlhäll CJ, Ebbers T, et al. 4D flow cardiovascular magnetic resonance consensus statement. *J Cardiovasc Magn Reson*. 2015;17(1):72.

[3]	Cheng HM, Lang D, Tufanaru C, Pearson A. Measurement accuracy of non-invasively obtained central blood pressure by applanation tonometry: a systematic review and meta-analysis. *International journal of cardiology*. 2013;167(5):1867-76.

[4]	Nelson MR, Stepanek J, Cevette M, Covalciuc M, Hurst RT, Tajik AJ. Noninvasive measurement of central vascular pressures with arterial tonometry: clinical revival of the pulse pressure waveform? *Mayo Clinic proceedings*. 2010;85(5):460-72.

[5]	O'Rourke MF. Vascular impedance in studies of arterial and cardiac function. *Physiological reviews*. 1982;62(2):570-623.

[6]	Hungerford SL, Adji AI, Bart NK, Lin L, Song N, Jabbour A, et al. Ageing, hypertension and aortic valve stenosis - Understanding the series circuit using cardiac magnetic resonance and applanation tonometry. *Int J Cardiol Hypertens*. 2021;9:100087.

[7]	Hungerford SL, Adji AI, Hayward CS, Muller DWM. Ageing, Hypertension and Aortic Valve Stenosis: A Conscious Uncoupling. *Heart Lung Circ*. 2021.

[8]	Qureshi MU, Colebank MJ, Schreier DA, Tabima DM, Haider MA, Chesler NC, et al. Characteristic impedance: frequency or time domain approach? *Physiol Meas*. 2018;39(1):014004.

[9]	Dujardin JP, Stone DN. Characteristic impedance of the proximal aorta determined in the time and frequency domain: a comparison. *Medical & biological engineering & computing*. 1981;19(5):565-8.

[10] Nichols WWR, M. F. Hartley, C. . *McDonalds Blood Flow in Arteries: Theoretical, experimental and clinical principles.*: Arnold and Oxford University Press Inc.; 1997.

[11] Mcdonald DA, Taylor MG, editors. *The Hydrodynamics of the Arterial Circulation* 1959.

[12] Womersley JR. Method for the calculation of velocity, rate of flow and viscous drag in arteries when the pressure gradient is known. *J Physiol.* 1955;127(3):553-63.

[13] Milnor WR. Arterial impedance as ventricular afterload. *Circulation research.* 1975;36(5):565-70.

[14] Nichols WW, Conti CR, Walker WE, Milnor WR. Input impedance of the systemic circulation in man. *Circulation research.* 1977;40(5):451-8.

[15] O'Rourke MF, Avolio AP. Pulsatile flow and pressure in human systemic arteries. Studies in man and in a multibranched model of the human systemic arterial tree. *Circulation research.* 1980;46(3):363-72.

[16] Murgo JP, Westerhof N, Giolma JP, Altobelli SA. Aortic input impedance in normal man: relationship to pressure wave forms. *Circulation.* 1980;62(1):105-16.

[17] Kelly R, Hayward C, Avolio A, O'Rourke M. Noninvasive determination of age-related changes in the human arterial pulse. *Circulation.* 1989;80(6):1652-9.

[18] Bollache E, Kachenoura N, Bargiotas I, Giron A, De Cesare A, Bensalah M, et al. How to estimate aortic characteristic impedance from magnetic resonance and applanation tonometry data? *Journal of hypertension.* 2015;33(3):575-82; discussion 83.

[19] Bargiotas I, Bollache E, Mousseaux E, Giron A, de Cesare A, Redheuil A, et al. MR and applanation tonometry derived aortic impedance: association with aging and left ventricular remodeling. *Journal of magnetic resonance imaging : JMRI.* 2015;41(3):781-7.

[20] Adji A, Kachenoura N, Bollache E, Avolio AP, O'Rourke MF, Mousseaux E. Magnetic resonance and applanation tonometry for noninvasive determination of left ventricular load and ventricular vascular coupling in the time and frequency domain. *Journal of hypertension.* 2016;34(6):1099-108.

[21] Namasivayam M, Adji A, Lin L, Hayward CS, Feneley MP, O'Rourke MF, et al. Non-Invasive Quantification of Ventricular Contractility, Arterial Elastic Function and Ventriculo-Arterial Coupling from a Single Diagnostic Encounter Using Simultaneous Arterial Tonometry and Magnetic Resonance Imaging. *Cardiovasc Eng Technol.* 2020;11(3):283-94.

[22] Beck DT, Martin JS, Nichols WW, Gurovich AN, Braith RW. Validity of a novel wristband tonometer for measuring central hemodynamics and augmentation index. *American journal of hypertension*. 2014;27(7):926-31.

[23] Hungerford SL, Adji AI, Bart NK, Lin L, Namasivayam MJ, Schnegg B, et al. A novel method to assess valvulo-arterial load in patients with aortic valve stenosis. *Journal of hypertension*. 2020.

[24] O'Rourke MF. Carotid Artery Tonometry: Pros and Cons. *American journal of hypertension*. 2016;29(3):296-8.

[25] Milnor WR, Bergel DH, Bargainer JD. Hydraulic power associated with pulmonary blood flow and its relation to heart rate. *Circulation research*. 1966;19(3):467-80.

[26] Milnor WR, Conti CR, Lewis KB, O'Rourke MF. Pulmonary arterial pulse wave velocity and impedance in man. *Circulation research*. 1969;25(6):637-49.

[27] Braunwald E, Gabe IT, Gault J, Mason DT, Mills CJ, Shillingford JP. Vascular impedance in man. *J Physiol*. 1969;202(1):10p.

[28] Murgo JP, Westerhof N. Input impedance of the pulmonary arterial system in normal man. Effects of respiration and comparison to systemic impedance. *Circulation research*. 1984;54(6):666-73.

[29] Freed BH, Collins JD, François CJ, Barker AJ, Cuttica MJ, Chesler NC, et al. MR and CT Imaging for the Evaluation of Pulmonary Hypertension. *JACC Cardiovascular imaging*. 2016;9(6):715-32.

[30] Gupta A, Sharifov OF, Lloyd SG, Tallaj JA, Aban I, Dell'italia LJ, et al. Novel Noninvasive Assessment of Pulmonary Arterial Stiffness Using Velocity Transfer Function. *Journal of the American Heart Association*. 2018;7(18):e009459.

[31] Ohyama Y, Redheuil A, Kachenoura N, Ambale Venkatesh B, Lima JAC. Imaging Insights on the Aorta in Aging. *Circulation Cardiovascular imaging*. 2018;11(4):e005617.

[32] Westerhof N, O'Rourke MF. Haemodynamic basis for the development of left ventricular failure in systolic hypertension and for its logical therapy. *Journal of hypertension*. 1995;13(9):943-52.

[33] Soulat G, Kachenoura N, Bollache E, Perdrix L, Diebold B, Zhygalina V, et al. *New estimate of valvuloarterial impedance in aortic valve stenosis: A cardiac magnetic resonance study. Journal of magnetic resonance imaging: JMRI*. 2017;45(3):795-803.

[34] Woldendorp K, Bannon PG, Grieve SM. Evaluation of aortic stenosis using cardiovascular magnetic resonance: a systematic review & meta-analysis. *Journal of cardiovascular magnetic resonance: official journal of the Society for Cardiovascular Magnetic Resonance*. 2020;22(1):45.

[35] Laskey WK, Kussmaul WG, 3rd. Hypertension, aortic valve stenosis, and the aorta: more lessons from TAVR. *Journal of the American College of Cardiology.* 2015;65(5):434-6.

[36] McLaughlin VV, Archer SL, Badesch DB, Barst RJ, Farber HW, Lindner JR, et al. ACCF/AHA 2009 expert consensus document on pulmonary hypertension: a report of the American College of Cardiology Foundation Task Force on Expert Consensus Documents and the American Heart Association: developed in collaboration with the American College of Chest Physicians, American Thoracic Society, Inc., and the Pulmonary Hypertension Association. *Circulation.* 2009;119(16):2250-94.

[37] Yotti R, Bermejo J, Gutierrez-Ibanes E, Perez del Villar C, Mombiela T, Elizaga J, et al. Systemic vascular load in calcific degenerative aortic valve stenosis: insight from percutaneous valve replacement. *Journal of the American College of Cardiology.* 2015;65(5):423-33.

[38] Ky B, French B, May Khan A, Plappert T, Wang A, Chirinos JA, et al. Ventricular-arterial coupling, remodeling, and prognosis in chronic heart failure. *Journal of the American College of Cardiology.* 2013;62(13):1165-72.

Contents of Earlier Volumes

Horizons in World Cardiovascular Research. Volume 18

Index